Occupational Therapy, Disability Activism, and Me

Occupational Therapy, Disability Activism, and Me

Challenging Ableism in Healthcare

GEORGIA VINE

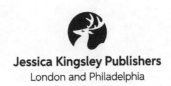

Jessica Kingsley Publishers
London and Philadelphia

First published in Great Britain in 2024 by Jessica Kingsley Publishers
An imprint of John Murray Press

2

Copyright © Georgia Vine 2024

The right of Georgia Vine to be identified as the Author of the Work has been
asserted by her in accordance with the Copyright, Designs and Patents Act 1988.

A CIP catalogue record for this title is available from the
British Library and the Library of Congress

ISBN 978 1 83997 667 4
eISBN 978 1 83997 668 1

Printed and bound in the United States by Integrated Books International

Jessica Kingsley Publishers' policy is to use papers that are natural,
renewable and recyclable products and made from wood grown in
sustainable forests. The logging and manufacturing processes are expected
to conform to the environmental regulations of the country of origin.

Jessica Kingsley Publishers
Carmelite House
50 Victoria Embankment
London EC4Y 0DZ

www.jkp.com

John Murray Press
Part of Hodder & Stoughton Ltd
An Hachette Company

With thanks to my mum, dad and sister Matilda,
for your continued support and love.

To Margaret and Georgina, this book wouldn't be possible without you.

Contents

Preface

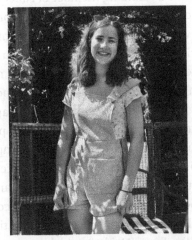

Image 0.1. *Georgia, a white female with dark curly hair, is standing outdoors. She has her sunglasses on her head and is wearing corded dungaree shorts and a top underneath, with flowers on.*

Hey! I'm Georgia, a disabled, white, cisgendered female with lived experience of cerebral palsy, and my pronouns are she/her. I am an occupational therapist and graduated with a first class honours degree in occupational therapy from Sheffield Hallam University in 2021.

Throughout my degree I developed my blog, *Not So Terrible Palsy*,[1] and it became more powerful than I could have ever imagined as it enabled me to analyse and contextualize my experiences as a disabled occupational therapy student. I did many series on my blog, a pivotal one being about my organically grown virtual placement during the second year of my degree in 2020. From this placement my blog grew, and I

---

1   https://notsoterriblepalsy.com

found that I had a platform within both the disabled community and the occupational therapy community – so much so that in the summer of 2020 I won the CP Teens UK[2] Upcoming Disability Blogger of the Year award. Having so much online growth and winning this award made me evaluate the content on my blog and how it was delivered. How could I keep on progressing? So I sharpened my activism tools and began to talk more openly about being a disabled occupational therapy student to critically evaluate my ableist experiences.

My passion for making an impact continued as my degree finalized, leading me to become a founding member of AbleOTUK.[3] AbleOTUK is a hub of advice, collaboration and peer support for those with health conditions, either within occupational therapy training or as graduates within the profession, and continues to be important to me.

After experiencing a huge delay in becoming a registered occupational therapist, my mental health was impacted and I felt the need to raise awareness of being both an occupational therapist and a disabled person. I wrote many guest blogs, which raised the profile of my work, and led to me gaining another accolade, becoming a Rising Star on the Shaw Trust Disability Power 100 list.[4] My content resonated with many readers, both disabled and non-disabled, and led me to give presentations at both national and international conferences. While writing this book, I was invited to present at the National Accessibility, Inclusion & Disability Expo (Naidex), which is a large event in the UK with over 8000 visitors.[5] This gave me the validation I desperately felt like I needed so early on in my career. My content actually had meaning that others could relate to and, most importantly, was making others question their own practice. This surprised me as I was initially utilizing my blog as a stream of consciousness to record my experiences as a disabled occupational therapist. To find that most of my experiences were universal was eye-opening and impactful, as I realized that my passion could also be my career.

Adding to this surprise, I also received a rather unexpected email from Jessica Kingsley Publishers in September 2021 about writing a book of my experiences. Me, writing a book? I am hugely passionate about

---

2   www.cpteensuk.org
3   https://affinot.co.uk/ableotuk
4   https://disabilitypower100.com
5   www.naidex.co.uk

blogging, but I never saw myself as a writer. I was never the best at English at school, and quite frankly still viewed my blogs as unstructured rambles. It never crossed my mind that they would make a good book or that I could ever be an author. But I was up for the challenge, and during the time that I put my book proposal together I began to really develop my passion for writing. I submitted my proposal in March 2022 and this solidified my goal of writing something that would be published to help my own mental health, never mind change the perceptions of others.

I knew that I could easily write about my experiences throughout my degree and my struggles to become a qualified occupational therapist. However, I was still questioning whether I could analyse my childhood experiences, as they were only those of one person, and so needed to be backed up by research and my knowledge gained from practice. Yes, I could write my stories and raise awareness, but I was longing for something deeper to connect my experiences to. When my proposal was accepted in April 2022 and I started writing the book, I was only a few months into my first job as a clinical demonstrator at the University of Huddersfield. Within this role I was a placement supervisor supporting occupational therapy students in their placements within a primary school, so I was carrying out research in this area. This led me to come across theories and research surrounding children's occupational therapy that backed up my blogs and life experience, validating my work and adding critical depth to my book. When the job finished in July, I had a few months between that and my next role, and I did nothing but write. I was so inspired by my work as a supervisor on a children's placement that I just kept writing about my childhood, and unpicking events that I had never intended to reflect on.

Writing this book then went from something that could be of interest to others to something that might start a very important conversation that many of us need to be having. My intention with the book is to create conversations and tangible action points that can be transferred to a wide variety of audiences. When I first experienced ableism, I thought it was just normal and accepted. Similarly, my own inner ableist voice quite often impacted my professional life as I felt the need to excel in order to 'prove' I was good enough as an activist and an occupational therapist. Looking through the lens of an occupational therapist as well as a disabled person, this book aims to question ableism within the integrated healthcare system. I acknowledge that this book only gives my own physical health perspective, and also tends to lean heavily on my occupational therapy background, but this is what my experiences cover, and it would be wrong of me to enter territory where I don't belong. However, I hope that the way this book is written means that such topics can still be interpreted by a variety of audiences including those with lived experience of disability, parents, teachers and other healthcare professionals.

Different people will get something different from reading this. Whether this alters your progress as an ally or as a fellow disabled person, we all need to continuously be learning from each other's experiences. If you can develop this further and apply some goals to your own life experiences with universal applicability, then please let me know!

I hope you enjoy reading this book and continue your journey towards #ChallengingAbleismInHealthcare. Please also fill out the 'Not So Terrible...P.A.L.S.Y.' reflective log after each chapter. The reflective log is there to help you contextualize your learning and start your allyship journey by setting future goals that challenge ableism and ableist structures.

PART ONE

Reflecting on My Childhood Experiences

CHAPTER ONE

Analysing My Diagnosis Through the Perspective of an Occupational Therapist and Disabled Activist

I'm in my early twenties and I have a publishing contract that I never would have received if I wasn't disabled. I'm pretty sure that I'm living my best disabled, chronically fabulous, life.

When I was younger, I, of course, had no perception of what disability was and what it meant, never mind ableism and disablism. As I've aged, my disability has become a bigger part of my identity. I know what you're thinking...hasn't it always been a part of your identity? Yes it has, but it's only in recent years that I have realized just how much my disability positively affects my identity and the role it plays in how I interpret everything around me. This skill has taken me a while to get the hang of, and is probably something I'll be forever trying to master. However, having the skillset of a disabled activist has made me analyse my life and look at it through a different lens, so throughout this book I will be using this skillset, as well as my own occupational therapy viewpoint, to highlight ableism within healthcare.

These first few chapters were the hardest to plan and write. Yes, it's hard to write chapters about stages of your life that you can barely remember. Emotionally it was much more challenging, as it made me realize how much ableism and disablism had been rooted in my life from the very beginning. But what is 'ableism' and 'disablism'? Scope defines ableism as 'discrimination in favour of non-disabled people' (Scope n.d.).

Ableism often results in disablism: 'Disablism refers to the ways in which people with impairments are disabled and disadvantaged by ableism's inequitable social structures and unjust practices' (Whalley Hammell 2022, p.1).

I experienced both of these when I was a young child, but it was never direct discrimination; it was simply because my disability was never accommodated due to society's 'inequitable social structure' (Whalley Hammell 2022, p.1). Nevertheless this discrimination was still there, and much of it was rooted in an approach that focused on what was 'wrong' with me rather than society's failings (Swaine 2011).

To find out more about the early stages of my diagnosis, I spoke to my parents **Glenda and Darron Vine.**

> **How was the diagnosis of my cerebral palsy delivered to you?**
>
> **Mum:** The delivery of the diagnosis was horrendous and very emotional. The appointment I was given said that you were going to see a physiotherapist. I was informed that they'd thought you'd had a stroke in the womb [there were other possible causes of my cerebral palsy, which I discuss later]. We went with your grandma who came to entertain Matilda [my younger sister] during the appointment. I walked in and, to my surprise, the consultant was also there. After a few assessments, I was given some distressing questions about my pregnancy. That's when the consultant bluntly said you had cerebral palsy, as simple as that. It was so overwhelming, I couldn't take it all in. I just got told you needed all this intense support from speech and language therapy, occupational therapy and physiotherapy, and that they would be in contact with us to develop a programme.
>
> The drive home was awful, with both your grandma and I crying due to the shock and anticipation. When you are in an emotional state and getting bombarded with information, you can't take it in. No thought or sensitivity was given to this delivery; I felt as if I was a number just going through a procedure, that was it. No person-centred practice was demonstrated.
>
> **Dad:** As I wasn't in the initial consultation, I found out through your mum, who I then had to console. I didn't really take this in, I was in a state of shock, and I knew your mum was unable to give me the full picture due to her distressing experience. I didn't have any

separate input; it was all through your mum. I only went to the main consultations due to the constraints of work. I felt like I was on the sidelines and no effort was made to look at us as a family.

What were your initial worries?

Mum: I was worried about your future. What the diagnosis entailed and what it meant for your life. I understand that cerebral palsy is an umbrella term and is different for everyone, but it's only through our experiences, knowing you, talking to others and seeking advice from the professionals ourselves that we've learned about CP [cerebral palsy]. We knew nothing back then, and I had to ask for this information from professionals to enhance my own knowledge rather than the knowledge being freely given to me.

Dad: I was scared as I didn't know what the outcome was going to be, and the minimal indication from the professionals didn't help either. I understand why so little information was given due to the variations of cerebral palsy, but the little communication given didn't help this process for us as a family. The lack of resources available for us to understand the scope of cerebral palsy and range of outcomes was also limited, resulting in more worry and confusion.

Did you receive any support?

Mum: Family supported us through this, and the professionals involved in your care were supportive once you started your regular programmes and they knew you more. This is when your support became more person-centred, yet it took a while to establish these relationships with the professionals.

I didn't have time to seek support elsewhere, such as attending parents' groups, as balancing work, life and all your medical appointments was difficult. Having chronic medical conditions myself, this made this balance even harder.

Dad: I didn't receive any support and felt like I had to support your mum, although neither of us knew what was going on. Family groups and organizations weren't easy to access for a working family; there was nothing local and nothing we could fit in to a busy family life.

When you started having your professional input, we felt more supported, but this was a slow build-up and wasn't very holistic.

How could this have been different?

Mum: More support from the very beginning, thinking about us as a family and our circumstances rather than just you. I felt neglected right from my pregnancy, and this only got worse with how much was expected from me just to be able to manage. I had to leave full-time employment when you were around 20 months old because I couldn't pursue my career due to not being able to commit. I got another job that was more suitable to our life; I did what any other mother would have done, but more support from professionals would have made this easier.

Dad: Working together as a team with the professionals to make sure your future journey was all-encompassing rather than just being passed among the different professionals. This was conflicting and left us confused when it came to knowing if your programme was individually tailored.

These are some very insightful answers from my parents about my diagnosis. I recognize that we are talking about a diagnosis that happened over 20 years ago and, although an ableist approach was clearly evident here, I want to understand more about diagnoses that happen currently. So I interviewed my cousin **Amanda Gaughan** whose son (my younger cousin and best pal), **Tommy Gaughan**, received a diagnosis of Down syndrome in 2018.

How was the diagnosis of Tommy's Down syndrome delivered to you?

Amanda: The screening was given with the blood test alongside the 12-week scan, and when this came back we received a phone call. One of the nurses called and said that we had a 1 in 30 'chance'. Further discussions were had regarding our options such as the amniocentesis test and the NIPT [non-invasive prenatal test], but at the time this wasn't available on the NHS [National Health Service] and we had to fund it privately. Also on the phone she said we had an option to not do anything or, if we wanted to terminate the pregnancy, we would have to take the amniocentesis. We were directed to a website called ARC (Antenatal Results and Choices).[1] On the phone I said I

---

1   www.arc-uk.org

just wanted to think about it, but the nurse called me back an hour later, worried about me.

ARC (Antenatal Results and Choices) is a government-endorsed website that provides links to information about antenatal screening, specific conditions or syndromes, and offers support with choices, loss and bereavement.

After a week, we decided to pay for the NIPT because amniocentesis has a resulting risk of miscarriage. We went to a private clinic and waited a week for the results to come back. When those results came back, the nurse called, telling us that she was very sorry that the result was positive for Down syndrome. She then asked if I was going to terminate or not. I didn't answer and asked to know the sex of our baby, which was included with the test, and she said 'it was a boy'. There was no further support offered, and we were told if we wanted more support to go back to a hospital.

We let the midwife at the hospital know our private test results and, by this point, we had decided we were keeping the baby. I had an appointment with a consultant and the screening midwife joined us. In that appointment, the consultant went through a long list of medical complications that Tommy may have and there was just one casual line at the end where he said that 'people with Down syndrome are living longer lives now'. He then asked if we still wanted to continue with our pregnancy and then he tried to push us to have the amniocentesis and I said no. They kept asking why, so I explained our worries about the risk of miscarriage, and how this wouldn't affect our decision anyway. So he tried to push the test again, saying that the chance of miscarriage was really low, to the point where I burst into tears and stated that I didn't want it.

The way that the diagnosis was shared has left a lasting negative impact on my emotional health.

What were your initial worries?
Amanda: Due to previous miscarriages I was worried about losing Tommy and I became very ill; these worries were only enhanced due

to stillbirth and other complications in Down syndrome pregnancies. I spoke to my midwife about it and she referred me to antenatal counselling. I was rejected from this service; following that, I became so ill that I was signed off work and my GP put a second successful referral in to the antenatal counselling service.

Other worries I had were about his health and if we would manage as a family with his extra needs. I worried whether I would be able to continue to work, about the impact on his siblings and what would happen to Tommy long term after we pass away. It was difficult to manage those considerations, which is why I joined online support groups.

Did you receive any support?
Amanda: The antenatal counselling wasn't specific to Down syndrome. The online support groups helped a lot, and now they offer so much more than what was available at the time I had Tommy. After he was born, we went to some Down syndrome support group meetings and met with other families. A parent representative also came to meet me while I was pregnant.

The support offered from the hospital directed us to support for additional testing and to terminating the pregnancy. During our consultant appointment, the screening midwife told us about the Down's Syndrome Association[2] but warned us they would present Down syndrome in an 'overly positive manner'.

The **Down's Syndrome Association** is a national organization promoting the rights and quality of life of individuals with Down syndrome.

What suggestions could you make to improve the service?
Amanda: The service needs to present a balanced view. Yes, share the potential health complications, but also share the real-life stories and present a balanced view so families can make an informed decision. Health professionals need to use neutral language; for

---

2   www.downs-syndrome.org.uk

example, the word 'chance' rather than 'risk' is better. There's now a sticker from Positive about Down syndrome[3] that can be placed on medical records so parents won't be continually asked about their decision throughout their pregnancy. I think hospitals should have an information pack available at screening for parents to look through. Parent representative details should be shared with you at the hospital during your screening so you can access that help quickly. Once you have had your screening, you are vulnerable and some will struggle to reach out due to heightened emotions and lack of time or energy due to being pregnant. Therefore, this information needs to be given as soon as possible to avoid any possible negative outcomes on mental health.

The antenatal counselling needs to have training for specific diagnoses. Positive about Down syndrome has counsellors who are experienced in parents who receive a Down syndrome diagnosis. They are available at a small cost through the charity. However, better signposting is still needed.

Positive about Down syndrome is a charity organization that provides stories to give parents, families and professionals a real picture of life with Down syndrome.

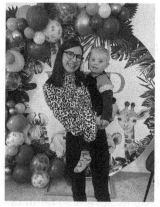

Image 1.1. *Georgia, a white female, holding her cousin Tommy, who is a white male toddler, on her hip. They have big grins and are surrounded by a balloon arch.*

---

3   https://positiveaboutdownsyndrome.co.uk

As shown from my parents and Amanda, the diagnosis led to a lot of *shock, worry* and *anticipation*, and understandably so. Any parent who has just been given a diagnosis for their child is going to worry about the medical complications that may arise, and I know that professionals have to present the possible range of scenarios. I'm in my twenties, and if I'm having a phase where my pain levels are higher than usual, I still worry even though I know it's just a flare up. We're all human! So imagine the worry a parent must face; every parent reacts differently, and this is okay.

Who knows what the future may entail? The fear of the unknown is worse, right? As my parents said, cerebral palsy is such an umbrella term, so when they (or rather Mum) got given the diagnosis, then of course they didn't know what to expect!

And if worrying about the future and medical complications isn't enough, parents have a whole new world to navigate. Even with my 20 plus years of experience, I'm still trying to figure out the world of disability. I love it, but it's a minefield. Imagine being unexpectedly thrown into this world with no preparation or expectation and with no guide on how to navigate it!

Scope has written a helpful article called 'Coming to terms with your child's diagnosis' (2022). This includes information and further signposting that can hopefully help you during this complex time.

Samantha Renke talks openly about the impact her diagnosis had on her family. Do read her book *You Are the Best Thing Since Sliced Bread* (2022). She also discusses her experiences being her unapologetic fabulous self, as she should be!

If you want to do some more research on diagnosis and what it means for you and your family, then do, especially if, like my parents and Amanda, you have been given very little information. However, this signposting should be provided from the professionals themselves, so seek this information from them, and check the source is reputable. For someone who's in a vulnerable position to start off with, diving into research can really be a mental strain – even if you know what you're doing there. Being certain about the reliability of a source is a minefield, even with the internet at our fingertips! Well, it's not at everyone's fingertips, and it certainly wasn't at my parents' fingertips in the early 2000s, so I guess that is the main difference between my and Tommy's diagnosis experience.

Worries for the future can permeate across parents and siblings too. When the bigger picture is revealed, the medical condition itself only plays a small part. As shown by the interviews in this book, healthcare professionals do not often consider this wider picture, resulting in systemic ableist repercussions and even worse outcomes for families.

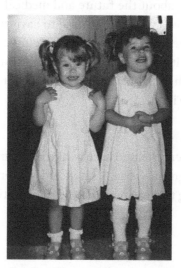

Image 1.2. *Two white female toddlers in dresses. My younger sister Matilda is on the left, and Georgia is on the right, wearing her AFOs (ankle foot orthoses).*

Amanda highlighted this when she spoke about how much impact Tommy's diagnosis had on her health. Of course it's going to affect her mental health. I am not a parent, so can't comment, but as an occupational therapist I know that physical and mental health are linked. It makes sense to suggest that this is the same concept for parents and carers carrying worries for their children.

Support for both my mum and Amanda was absent from the beginning, and both felt neglected, even during pregnancy. As a result of the complications my mum faced during pregnancy I was born five weeks premature and was additionally then starved of oxygen at birth, resulting in my cerebral palsy. Meaning, if my mum's physical health hadn't been compromised, I may never have been born with cerebral palsy and might not have been here writing this book today. Not that we would have it any other way now, but talk about the lack of person-centred practice!

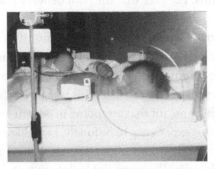

Image I.3. *Georgia, a white baby, in an incubator, connected to machinery while sleeping.*

The process in both these cases was thoughtless, with a scarcity of information. Why aren't different professionals working with families collaboratively from the start? I understand that consultants are not trained to draw on their therapeutic use of self like occupational therapists are, but there are times when that empathy is needed. The 'intentional relationship model' defines the therapeutic self as applying unique interpersonal characteristics to understand an individual on an interpersonal level (Taylor 2020). I hope that both my and Tommy's diagnoses would have been delivered differently if an occupational therapist had been in the room.

Both my parents highlighted the need for multidisciplinary involvement, which wasn't a shock to me. This is clearly an important factor to my parents as they felt it was missing at the point of diagnosis. How daunting must it feel for your family to get passed from professional to professional rather than having everyone in the same meeting? To be fair, cerebral palsy is an umbrella term and no one can predict the future, but surely a holistic team should be established on receiving that diagnosis. Maybe this is done now, and I'd hope delivery of diagnosis is done a lot better than it was in the early 2000s, but here's one thing I do know as an occupational therapist: working as a multidisciplinary team is vital. I've studied the importance of interprofessional working at university, I've read the reports and seen the distressing stories where this wasn't the case. This means that this interprofessional support should be there right from diagnosis in order to offer the best support for families.

Diagnosis is, of course, going to impact families no matter how this news is given, as people have feelings. From interviewing both my parents and Amanda, I can see that the poor delivery made the outcome much worse.

Although internet access and online communities are essential to community-building and discovering information, some people don't have access to the internet. At the time of my diagnosis, many of these groups met in person and there wasn't this sense of online community. My parents' busy lives meant that attending in person was difficult, so at times they found this experience to be lonely. I would really recommend exploring relevant online communities because, believe me, they are not 'overly positive' places (as the nurse dubbed them to Amanda). They are places filled with pure joy, and it is a privilege to be a part of them. Heck, everyone needs the beauty of the disabled community in their lives.

Physical health impacts on self-esteem, therefore affecting mental health (Creek *et al.* 2022). I acknowledge my bias and my experiences having been around physical health, yet there are times when my mental health has been impacted by my disability. The disabled community is particularly important to me, as it's a world where I can just be myself. Ableism and oppression is not easy to deal with and gets internalized within the family even before a child is born, when the disabled individual is viewed as a 'burden' and a 'tragedy' (David 2013, p.7):

> Internalized oppression is not the cause of our mistreatment; it is the result of our mistreatment. It would not exist without the real external oppression that forms the social climate in which we exist. Once oppression has been internalized...the pain and the memories, the fears and the confusions, the negative self-images and the low expectations [begin]. (Marks 1999, cited in Kumari Campbell 2009, p.25)

This is why I *had* to interview Amanda about Tommy's diagnosis. The words 'it was a boy' were given in the past tense, as if the baby was no longer a current event, referred to with an impersonal 'it' pronoun... seriously? It frustrates me that this still happens in practice; you don't have to be a disabled activist to see how wrong this statement is! This is microaggression at its finest, which again contributes to internalized ableism, gaslighting and the projection of pity: 'Microaggression occurs as intangible discriminating and prejudiced interactions, whether intentional or unintentional' (David 2013, p.2).

I knew that writing this chapter would be difficult, but it's been a lot more emotional than I thought. When you're in the whirlwind of having a disability, you don't have time to stop, think and analyse. I never complained about being in children's services as a child, and we, as a family, thought that the service we received was top-notch. Even when it came to receiving this diagnosis, my parents didn't have time to analyse it as it was unalterable and they had to get ready to fight the next battle. Analysing this experience now, it has taken its toll on both my parents and myself, as we now know that my time in children's services was far from top-notch. It's difficult to accept that, and I don't want people who are reading this book to think that I am a negative person – as actually my life is amazing, and I wouldn't change a thing (except for the ableist systems).

We must break this stigma around diagnosis, but to do this we have to address the ableism and disablism that is projected onto healthcare systems by wider societal barriers and attitudes, such as the way that societal attitudes view disability, as if it's something to be pitied, or that I, as a disabled person, can be 'cured' by yoga, for example. My life is not something to be pitied, I don't need to be 'cured', and I am certainly not a burden! I'm in my early twenties and I have a publishing contract that I never would have received if I wasn't disabled. I'm pretty sure that I'm living my best disabled, chronically fabulous, life. Those outside of the world of disability don't see the pure joy that comes with the disabled life and our community; they just focus solely on the 'deficits' and what someone 'can't do' rather than their strengths and possibilities. This leads to low expectations and negativity, and we must change the record.

So what do you think could be done to ensure diagnosis is holistic and not just focused on 'deficits'?

NOT SO TERRIBLE...P.A.L.S.Y. REFLECTIVE LOG

Pausing

Stop and think about what you have read in this chapter. What are your main takeaway points? What are your main questions?

....

....

....

Analysing

Why did this resonate with you?

....

....

....

Learning

What did you learn from this?

....

....

....

Solving

What actions need to be put into place?

....

....

....

Your plan

How will you achieve these actions? What are your goals?

....

....

....

References

Creek, J., Bryant, W., Fieldhouse, J. and Bannigan, K. (2022) *Creek's Occupational Therapy and Mental Health* (6th edn). Glasgow: Elsevier Health.

David, E.J.R. (2013) *Internalised Oppression: The Psychology of Marginalised Groups.* New York: Springer Publishing Company.

Kumari Campbell, F. (2009) 'Internalised Ableism: The Tyranny Within.' In F. Kumari Campbell, *Contours of Ableism: The Production of Disability and Abledness* (pp.16–29). London: Palgrave Macmillan.

Marks, D. (1999) *Disability: Controversial Debates and Psychosocial Perspectives.* London: Routledge.

Renke, S. (2022) *You Are the Best Thing Since Sliced Bread.* London: Penguin Books. Accessed on 31 March 2023 at www.penguin.co.uk/books/447975/you-are-the-best-thing-since-sliced-bread-by-renke-samantha/9781529149289

Scope (2022) 'Coming to terms with your child's diagnosis.' Accessed on 19 August 2022 at www.scope.org.uk/advice-and-support/come-to-terms-with-child-diagnosis

Scope (no date) 'Disablism and ableism.' Accessed on 30 May 2022 at www.scope.org.uk/about-us/disablism

Swaine, Z. (2011) 'Medical Model.' In J.S. Kreutzer, J. DeLuca and B. Caplan (eds) *Encyclopedia of Clinical Neuropsychology* (pp.1542–1543). New York: Springer. Accessed on 18 March 2023 at https://doi.org/10.1007/978-0-387-79948-3_2131

Taylor, R. (2020) *The Intentional Relationship Model: Occupational Therapy and Therapeutic Use of Self.* United States: F.A. Davis Company.

Whalley Hammell, K. (2022) 'Editorial: Occupational therapy and the right to occupational participation.' *Irish Journal of Occupational Therapy 50*, 1, 1–2. Accessed on 3 August 2022 at https://doi.org/10.1108/IJOT-05-2022-031

CHAPTER TWO

Reflecting on My Time in Children's Services

I must have had so much internalized ableism to believe that an activity that most kids that age do was too costly to adapt for my needs.

The medical model of disability suggests that disability is identified through systematic processes such as tests and examinations, and a major weakness of the model is that it focuses on a person's inabilities (Swaine 2011). Ding! Ding! Ding! Ring any bells? In the previous chapter I explored how medicalized my cerebral palsy and my cousin Tommy's Down syndrome diagnoses were, and the low expectations forced on us by medical professionals. Why is the world so focused on what we *can't* do rather than embracing our beautiful differences? This is really important to recognize if you use standardized assessments in any area.

Reflecting on our views is essential. I hold my hand up, however, as I know that I've been ableist myself, and have taken inspiration from those with disabilities who are performing everyday activities. I have teared up from videos of poor children in the pity parades that you see in the media. But it's important to critically explore why we think in certain ways.

We all have people who inspire us, regardless of who we are and where we come from, whether this be a parent or carer, teacher or a public figure. However, do we ever stop and think about why these people actually become our role models? Fellow activists inspire me with their ideas as they make me think *critically* about how I see the world, making me question my thoughts. But they do not inspire me solely because they get up and go to work. Okay, maybe disabled activists do inspire me a little through doing these activities as I can personally relate to their fatigue and their struggles against an ableist society. 'Inspiration porn' is a term used by Stella Young in her TEDx Talk (2014) to refer to disabled people being objectified in order to make non-disabled people feel better about themselves morally. So if you can't relate personally to my experiences, then I shouldn't be your muse.

Healthcare professionals working in rehabilitation are guided by the biomedical model of disability, seeing disability as a 'problem' to be 'fixed' (Yao *et al.* 2022). Yao *et al.*'s must-read research analyses how the occupational therapy profession sees disability as something that needs intervention, ignoring societal issues, injustices and accessibility. This is why society often sees disability as the problem and not the ableist environment that limits the disabled person.

When exploring Scope's definition of ableism, the phrase that stuck out to me was *in favour of non-disabled people* (Scope n.d.) as this is what it has felt like my whole life. Society and cultural norms are built to favour non-disabled people, and this makes navigating disabled life so much more complex.

The social model of disability argues that it is the barriers in society that disable people and not their impairments (Oliver 2013). For example, I am disabled because of environmental barriers such as limited access and people's attitudes towards cerebral palsy rather than my CP itself. Reflecting on the ableist experiences in my life, I agree, and I've felt more disabled as I've aged due to facing more barriers. Before I started school I didn't feel 'disabled' because society doesn't judge if a toddler falls over or needs more support with physical activity. However, I now realize that the 'norm' doesn't consider me.

The cultural model understands that everyone's experience of disability is independent (Waldschmidt 2017), so it's understandable that this book only explores my experiences rather than generalized answers. This is why it's so important to listen to different disabled people and to learn from us. The social model cannot be applied to all cultures, which is something we need to consider when addressing systemic ableism. Political and cultural values give us a deeper understanding of how disability is viewed differently (Waldschmidt 2017). This makes me think about how cultural factors are considered in some of the different occupational therapy models. However, some of these lack a holistic overview since they are based on systemic injustices and possible cultural biases themselves. Do you sense the vicious cycle here?

The World Federation of Occupational Therapists (WFOT) refers to occupation as 'the everyday activities that people do as individuals, in families and with communities to occupy time and bring meaning and purpose to life. Occupations include things people need to, want to and are expected to do' (WFOT 2018). My memories of children's services are filled with working towards the activities of daily living (ADLs) that it seems we are socially obligated to participate in. Yao *et al.*'s research explores how certain ADLs are seen as compulsory, 'as if a hierarchy of occupations exist' (Yao *et al.* 2022, p.7), with self-care occupations such as washing and dressing often being prioritized. Yet this fails to acknowledge health considerations and dehumanizes those who have an alternative daily routine. Furthermore, a child's preferences may be ignored as that meaningful occupation a child may want to prioritize may come further down in the adults' priority list.

One joyful memory that I can recall during my time in children's services was getting my trike funded by the Royal Variety Charity. Oh, I was over the moon when the physiotherapist asked what the main goal was that I'd love to work towards as she mentioned my desire to ride a bike. This was such an exciting process from beginning to end, even for my parents, especially when Frazer Hines from *Emmerdale Farm* rocked up at my door to announce that I had received funding. Of course, my sister and I had no idea who he was at age eight/nine, and were probably very disappointed that it wasn't Miley Cyrus.

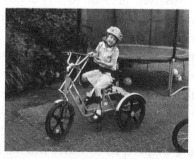

Image 2.1. *Georgia, a white female, as a child on her pink trike in the garden. A trampoline is behind. She is wearing her school dress and has a helmet on (even the helmet is a Hannah Montana helmet, so you can tell she was definitely a fan of Miley Cyrus).*

Due to this experience and many more, I did enjoy my appointments in children's services (I guess I had always been a budding occupational therapist from a young age). However, when the physiotherapist asked me what I wanted to achieve I was taken aback as I'd never been asked that question before. Riding a bike had quickly come to mind, yet I didn't think it was possible as it wasn't an essential occupation. I was amazed – my physiotherapist read my mind! I must have had so much internalized ableism to believe that an activity that most kids that age do was too costly to adapt for my needs.

It was ingrained in me to just work towards those essential ADLs and to do standardized assessment after standardized assessment. I understand that some things come with practice and I did need to improve my fine motor skills, otherwise I might not be sat here typing today (other access methods are out there but are used less frequently as they cost more, both financially and in terms of energy). Yet, looking back now, constantly being assessed and being told that I didn't fit in a box just doesn't make sense.

To bring in an even more experienced perspective on standardized assessments, I interviewed **Dr Benita Powrie** who has been working in paediatrics around the world for over 25 years.

How ableist are standardized assessments?
Benita: Many standardized assessments are inherently ableist. Developmental assessments or assessments of performance components actively position the person against the 'norm'. The 'norm' of what is expected is set by testing the assessment on large numbers of 'normal' children, actively excluding disabled children.

Standardized assessments are often then misused, and people with disabilities are particularly impacted by this – such as using developmental assessments and milestones developed with non-disabled children. For example, using IQ testing on young people with cerebral palsy is highly likely to misrepresent a child's abilities as the test was not designed to accommodate different motor skills, yet this does still occur.

Why do we still use standardized assessments as the 'gold standard'?
Benita: Different standardized assessments, used appropriately and as designed, can help to identify where developmental differences are emerging, measure change or uncover what parts of the occupation

are problematic. But assessing for assessments' sake to build a picture of deficits does not aid in decision-making and can be quite damaging to children and families. They also use a lot of time and resources.

However, standardized assessments, like the Family Goal-Setting Tool (FGST),[1] developed alongside families, is a good resource. As long as we are working with families to help identify goals together, we are using good practice.

Standardized assessments can have a place in helping to identify issues that can be addressed. For example, blood tests or early identification of cerebral palsy...using the General Movements Assessment[2] can lead to effective interventions that can improve quality of life.

The **Family Goal Setting Tool (FGST)** is a card-sorting exercise for healthcare professionals and teachers who work with children and their families. It helps prioritize individual and family needs and goals.

The **General Movements Assessment** is a cost-effective, non-invasive assessment that identifies neurological patterns, and could lead to an early diagnosis of cerebral palsy and other developmental disabilities.

What message does standardized assessments give to children and parents?

Benita: Historically, in my own practice parents and children were given messages about deficits, problems and differences. Although this was done with good intention, it was following a mechanist reductive medical model approach that I fear may have done more harm than good for some. Time spent focusing on what you *can't*

---

1   https://autismqld.com.au/resources/the-family-goal-setting-tool-fgst
2   https://cerebralpalsy.org.au/our-research/about-cerebral-palsy/what-is-cerebral-palsy/signs-and-symptoms-of-cp/general-movements-assessment

do takes away from what you *can* do. Such an approach risked reinforcing to the parents that their child was disabled in some way or was 'less than', and there are ways we could have done that better.

Should we, as healthcare professionals, be challenging the use of these assessments?

Benita: I think we absolutely should be thinking very carefully about the assessments we use and why. Our understanding of development, occupational performance and what works in terms of interventions has changed significantly. Therefore, our *bottom-up performance, component-based standardized assessments should not have a place in practice*. Assessments that help understand context, performance of valued occupations and people's aspirations and goals fit much better with our current evidence-based practice, as well as being more respectful and person-centred.

Whatever assessments we use, we need to think carefully about how we make sure someone can give informed consent. Do parents, carers and young people understand the implications of this assessment?

Standardized or non-standardized, the feelings around being assessed never go away; there is always that fear of being judged, especially when the assessor is someone you've never met. So many worries and questions go through your mind. Will they have read my notes before meeting me and have preconceived ideas of me and my situation? Or will they have not read anything, leaving it up to me to retell my personal and often traumatic information yet again? It's a very fine line. I understand that assessments are needed and, when done successfully, can lead to great outcomes, but it's still daunting, and this then affects performance. I remember once being asked to count down in sevens from 100; at the time I'd just applied to study A-Level maths at college, I loved it! Yet the pressure of that situation affected my performance, and this was even within my natural home environment.

A lot of questions from both Benita and myself came out of the interview, such as: do standardized assessments contribute towards diagnoses? Do they measure change? Do they help with working towards achievement of goals?

Those who use children's services may be too young or have

disabilities that impact on them understanding the full scope of any assessments they're given. My cousin **Amanda Gaughan** has gone through many assessments with her son **Tommy** who has Down syndrome, so I asked her about my queries in an interview.

> **What are both your and Tommy's experiences of assessments, and what is their value to you as a family?**
> **Amanda:** The assessments that they offer are for 'typical' children, so they were meaningless for Tommy. He used the *Development Journal for Babies and Children with Down Syndrome*,[3] which was much more meaningful as it showed how well Tommy was doing. Yet there is such a wide variety in ability in children with Down syndrome, therefore you can't presume that all areas of development will be delayed. The only value of the assessments to us is that you have to be assessed in order to gain access to support or equipment.
>
> Most appointments require travel and can be lengthy. This has impacted on my other son. Most health professionals have been wonderful, but occasionally there are some who use outdated language, which can be offensive.

The **Council for Disabled Children**[4] is a charity that works towards inclusion within education, health and social care. They provide early support for children and their families. Their resource, the *Development Journal for Babies and Children with Down Syndrome*, is given to monitor early progress and learning.

Many standardized tests are overly medicalized, which, as Amanda mentioned, is not only offensive and outdated for service users, it is also difficult for families. If a parent has been told that their child needs an assessment, then of course they'll give consent. But often, as Benita points out, young people and families don't understand the implications and can't predict how useful the assessment will be. Yes, of course some assessments will have to be done as a starting point for investigations.

---

3   https://councilfordisabledchildren.org.uk/resources/all-resources/filter/schools-colleges-and-fe/downs-syndrome-development-journal-early
4   https://councilfordisabledchildren.org.uk

But we need to make sure that we are not assessing for the sake of it, as this is unfair on families trying to navigate what is already a complicated world.

Although I believe that standardized assessments stem from ableist practices, using assessments such as the Family Goal-Setting Tool (FGST) means that the whole family can make holistic goals as a unit. So it would be very ignorant of me to sit here and say that all standardized assessments are ableist as some can have a powerful impact. Getting a diagnosis is another example that can be a great, validating experience for some, giving access to services and support.

Other assessments aren't as useful, however, and it's sad that some compare disabled children against the 'norms' of non-disabled children in order for them to gain access to support, enabling them to receive what are basic human rights. The phrase 'set up for failure' comes to mind. Again, these approaches play a huge role in why disability has such a negative perception for other people. How are families who are new to the world of disability meant to view this in a positive light when these ableist views are constantly being perpetuated? It can be so damaging to families to focus on the negatives and 'inabilities' to gain access to any support. I'm grateful for my wheelchair, but movement is a human right, and I need that wheelchair to function in society with reduced pain and fatigue.

Outcome measures need to be evaluated and we need to critically look at the labelling used. Labels may measure disability in terms of 'good', 'fair' or 'poor', but this is based on the therapist's subjective opinion (Yao *et al.* 2022). If an occupational therapist was to observe me sweating while making my bed, they may not see this as 'good', yet it wouldn't matter to me. I've found my adapted way to do this and I'm going to stick to it. Yes, there are risks involved but, as occupational therapists, we know that we can't eliminate all risks and have to enable positive risk taking. Yet healthcare support is often focused on 'fixing' perceived weaknesses rather than viewing the person as a whole. Everyone's perception of 'quality of life' is different, and of course a disabled person's quality of life is going to differ from a non-disabled person's (Yao *et al.* 2022), but this does not mean it is of lesser importance. I struggle to style my hair; yes, some days it's frustrating, but I don't aspire to be a hairdresser, so it's not affecting my quality of life. We need to be continually asking ourselves whether we are assessing what's meaningful to the person.

Intervention should be collaborative, although there is a chance professionals coerce individuals into choosing the occupation that meets their progress towards a perceived need to 'normalize', thus failing to acknowledge that individuals are experts in their own lives (Yao *et al.* 2022). For example, I was given weighted cutlery to reduce my jerky movements, yet the pain that it caused me was actually more disruptive than the jerky movements themselves. Yes, some days I do get food everywhere, but we all have good days and bad days, right?

Another example is that my handwriting was not legible regardless of the amount of interventions that I was given, so I had a feeling that it was never going to be legible. It still isn't, just to clarify, even in my twenties; I still have to decipher what I've written in someone's birthday card, so don't take it personally if I only write 'Love Georgia x' – well, that's if you can read it, of course! Typing is my preference anyway as handwriting causes me pain. I'm not going to deny the fact that there were times where I did want to work on my handwriting. However, the main reason for my reluctance was that when interventions focused on this, we worked *towards* handwriting but rarely worked on the handwriting itself.

Even when therapy is person-centred, lots of time is spent focusing on the individual components that combine to form an occupation or action. This is because every goal is so focused on being *'able to'* (Yao *et al.* 2022, p.8), but *'able'* reinforces professional power, actively promoting ableism (Whalley Hammell 2022). For example, 'for Georgia to be *able to* write her name using a tripod grip', using the bottom-up approach, I would have to work on other components such as grip, strength and hand–eye coordination. But through using a top-down approach to assess my writing skill, you might find that I may never be able to use a tripod grip, despite this causing less pain and stress on the body for a 'normal' person. Actually, I do write using a tripod grip, but if the practitioners just let me write during interventions, they would realize I just needed repeated practice to work towards legibility.

I understand that for some occupations, certain components do need to be worked on first – just like you wouldn't run a marathon without training. But there are multiple ways to perform an occupation, and it doesn't matter if it's achieved in the same way as the 'norm' would.

This is why I love evidence-based practice because we can explore new interventions and strategies. As occupational therapists, we can keep up to date with research to better our own practice and services. When the first solution doesn't work, we need to provide a safe space to prevent disheartenment and continue to explore other methods to achieve that occupation.

My awareness of disability began in nursery, but the gap became more apparent at school, and more provisions and support were required. I could perform the occupations that my peers could do – I just did things differently. There are aids I still use today and was given at a young age by occupational therapists, such as my plate guard, which is a raised ring that surrounds my dinner plate to stop food sliding off as I eat. However, there are some occupations my family and I had to find creative solutions for ourselves. Let's use the classically evaluated occupation of making a cup of tea. When I make a cup of tea, after pouring the water onto the teabag, I carry it to the table before grabbing the milk; this ensures the cup isn't full when I'm carrying it. Disabled people are certainly gurus at creating innovative solutions!

This statement from Whalley Hammell sums it up perfectly, saying that this way of bodily function-focused practice is ableist. Hey, I'm not calling you ableist if you're a paediatric occupational therapist, but unfortunately the systems can be: 'Ableist values shape the practices of occupational therapists, such that patients are exhorted to minimize their bodily deviations from the dominant group's valued norms, strive to attain higher levels of physical function, achieve independence in self-care and become more productive' (Whalley Hammell 2022-a, p.1).

The same goes for school. As a disabled child, I was disadvantaged as soon as I started school by being pushed to meet a National Curriculum that was based on the standards of the non-disabled population. For example, I know from my practice within a school that at age five a child is expected to run, jump, hop and climb, but that doesn't consider disabled pupils. I didn't meet those milestones at that age, and still struggle with some of those activities 20 years later. As an occupational therapy educator during a placement at a school, I demonstrated these actions to the university students, and the four- and five-year-olds certainly had more balance than I did!

There is so much systemic ableism in schools, and disabled children are often not enabled to thrive. Without realizing it, this had a massive effect on me, and deeply rooted many forms of internalized ableism, which was enhanced further by all the drawn-out unexpected battles I faced. My parents recognized that the education system was unfair from the beginning, and so they fought hard to put into place my Education, Health and Care Plan (EHCP), or what was called a 'Statement' back then.

How did you find out about EHCPs?

Mum: It was a parent who said, 'Are you going for a Statement for Georgia?' At the time, I had no idea what this was and had to then research. From research, I knew it was what you needed to achieve your full potential. The National Curriculum is wrong; I always knew it wasn't fair that you were being assessed on the same scale as everyone else; it's ableist.

Dad: I found out through your mum who did the research, information on this was very limited and at the time we felt very alone.

What was the process?

Mum: It took years. I had to collate a magnitude of reports and evidence from school and healthcare professionals – it was a very anxiety-provoking process. Constantly chasing everyone and arranging interdisciplinary meetings didn't help either. Trying to attend these meetings as a family was near enough impossible while working and looking after two young children. Arranging time off of work constantly had a mental strain, and I was worried about being penalized or potentially losing my job.

Then, when you finally got the Statement, I had to appeal because of the measly hours that you were offered for one-to-one support as these were insufficient to enable you to achieve your full potential. I had no other option but to see my local MP, who was David Blunkett at the time. This sped up the appeal and, after years of being mentally and physically drained, we won our appeal.

Dad: Your mum took the leading role to gather information and arranged all of the meetings needed to facilitate the Statement. After the initial offering of limited support, your mum contacted Citizens Advice and arranged a meeting with the local MP who was an ally as he was registered as being blind. He was 100 per cent on our side to increase the support to help you achieve your highest academic potential.

How easy was it to get the support we needed?
Mum: We had to fight for everything. It was an extremely long-winded process due to the amount of red tape that we faced; this put a lot of pressure on our family dynamic.

Dad: It was very difficult as there was no specific process already in place, so everything was hard to find and even harder to accomplish.

What support did we receive?
Mum: School was really supportive and the healthcare professionals backed us up all the way. Our wider family helped a lot in terms of supporting us. I felt I had to shout the loudest just to be listened to and, even then, that meant waiting for weeks on end to receive a phone call or receive the letters that we needed.

I registered you as disabled and joined the Sheffield Parent Carer Forum, which helped me a lot with signposting. I received their leaflets and booklets through the post, which enabled me to communicate effectively with professionals when having important discussions.

Dad: School accepted the Statement with open arms as it increased your support to help you attain higher and better results. We had to rely heavily on family and friends to aid our attendance of meetings. Our support network provided the space we needed to fight for everything.

What could be different?
Mum: The education and the awareness back then was non-existent and no signposting was given. The access to resources was poor and it took a long time to delve through physical sources of information. I needed to be more informed so I could do my best as a parent for our family. I only found about Disability Living Allowance because your grandma spotted a leaflet while waiting for a physiotherapy appointment.

Dad: This system should have been integrated in terms of communication between children's services and your school. We only found out about other support systems through third parties, whereas we should have found out from the professionals themselves. There's no education on the aid that is out there; when you're a young family who have never dealt with the world of disability, it is challenging.

Let's start by looking at the fact that my parents had to be the ones who instigated my EHCP. I hope that the integrated care system is a lot more prepared and accessible now than it was 20 years ago. Why isn't this complicated process broken down for families? Why isn't everything you need to know about EHCPs provided as an educational resource?

We didn't even find out about Disability Living Allowance through healthcare professionals. Living with a disability comes with a huge price increase, with disabled people facing an average cost of an extra £975 a month compared to non-disabled people, and £1248 if there are two disabled members of the household (Scope n.d.-a), so families need to know about available financial support!

Read **Scope**'s useful page on the extra costs of disability to find out about the financial help you may be eligible for (Scope n.d.-a).

Even after starting this process, the foreseeable future will often be filled with long-winded red tape. I understand that, due to waiting times, a process like this cannot be done overnight, but my mum shouldn't have had to chase up so many things. This is such a complicated process and the care system should have been integrated! Families shouldn't be put through this exhausting and anxiety-provoking process.

Of course support and aid cost money; this is a political concern, and not just ableism. But families shouldn't be made anxious or have to worry about job security, which puts a strain on the family dynamic. Again, this needs to be looked at holistically by the integrated care system. Surely better support systems can be put in place that guide families through this process without it weighing so heavily on their lives?

Even when my educational support was agreed, we had to appeal and get our local MP involved. We are so fortunate that at the time our local MP was David Blunkett, because he was highly informed about the process and understood a disabled perspective. This comes back to listening to disabled voices because we have lived experience of disability and know our stuff!

Getting my EHCP was when we, as a family, realized how many fronts you have to put on when living with a disability. You spend half of your life almost downplaying your disability so that society recognizes you as a valuable individual. Yet the other half of our time is spent recalling our worst symptoms in order to receive the support needed. This juggling act is still an ongoing battle that I face. No wonder it was so hard for my parents at this time.

Once I was granted a more reasonable EHCP, my one-to-one learning began with the most wonderful lady. There genuinely aren't enough words to describe how much love I have for that support assistant – I am very grateful and thankful for all of her support to enable me to get where I am today. My time in education really did change for the better when my one-to-one was put into place as I finally had the support I needed. I do have good memories of school and I always enjoyed going to school. One time, my teacher taped the egg to the spoon in the egg and spoon race as they knew I couldn't balance the egg on the spoon without this aid. I became smug and started to run, but within a few paces the egg was dangling from the spoon on the tape!

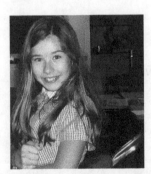

Image 2.2. *Georgia, a white female, aged ten, who is sat smiling at school in the classroom.*

I was just a number to the schooling system; because of this attitude, disabled children are still not always pushed to thrive. For example, maths had always been my strong point and I was always in the top class. I took pride in this as I was often reduced to my disability elsewhere. But due to my inability to handwrite, telling my support assistant how to lay out mathematical equations on the page was tough, so I often took longer to do the work. As a result, my teachers in primary school wanted to move me down into the lower level class. In the end, I remained in the top class, but this shows how ableist the schooling system was, and this awareness is what mainstream schools lack – no creative thought is given to enable disabled children to achieve targets in their own way.

My cerebral palsy meant that I had to overcome many barriers. I still managed to achieve my goals in life through finding innovative solutions where needed. I shouldn't have been met with so many issues from an early age, including the overly macrocosmic standardized assessments, and the fight my family experienced to put reasonable adjustments in place within the school system.

NOT SO TERRIBLE...P.A.L.S.Y. REFLECTIVE LOG
Pausing
Stop and think about what you have read in this chapter. What are your main takeaway points? What are your main questions?

. . . .

. . . .

. . . .

Analysing
Why did this resonate with you?

. . . .

. . . .

. . . .

Learning
What did you learn from this?

. . . .

. . . .

. . . .

Solving
What actions need to be put into place?

....

....

....

Your plan
How will you achieve these actions? What are your goals?

....

....

....

References

Oliver, M. (2013) 'The social model of disability: Thirty years on.' *Disability & Society* 28, 7, 1024–1026. Accessed on 18 March 2023 at www.tandfonline.com/doi/full/10.1080/09687599.2013.818773?needAccess=true

Scope (no date) 'Disablism and ableism.' Accessed on 30 May 2022 at www.scope.org.uk/about-us/disablism

Scope (no date-a) 'Disability Price Tag 2023: The extra cost of disability.' Accessed on 24 July 2023 at www.scope.org.uk/campaigns/extra-costs/disability-price-tag-2023

Swaine, Z. (2011) 'Medical Model.' In J.S. Kreutzer, J. DeLuca and B. Caplan (eds) *Encyclopedia of Clinical Neuropsychology* (pp.1542–1543). New York: Springer. Accessed on 18 March 2023 at https://doi.org/10.1007/978-0-387-79948-3_2131

Waldschmidt, A. (2017) 'Disability Goes Cultural. The Cultural Model of Disability as an Analytical Tool.' In A. Waldschmidt, H. Berressem and M. Ingwersen (eds) *Culture – Theory – Disability* (pp.19–28). Bielefeld: transcript Verlag. Accessed on 21 September 2022 at https://doi.org/10.14361/9783839425336-003

WFOT (World Federation of Occupational Therapists) (2018) 'Definitions of Occupational Therapy from Member Organisations.' Accessed on 13 June 2022 at www.wfot.org/resources/definitions-of-occupational-therapy-from-member-organisations

Whalley Hammell, K. (2022) 'A call to resist occupational therapy's promotion of ableism.' *Scandinavian Journal of Occupational Therapy.* Accessed on 1 January 2023 at https://doi.org/10.1080/11038128.2022.2130821

Whalley Hammell, K. (2022-a) 'Editorial: Occupational therapy and the right to occupational participation.' *Irish Journal of Occupational Therapy 50*, 1, 1–2. Accessed on 3 August 2022 at https://doi.org/10.1108/IJOT-05-2022-031

Yao, D.P.G., Sy, M.P., Martinez, P.G.V. and Laboy, E.C. (2022) 'Is occupational therapy an ableist health profession? A critical reflection on ableism and occupational therapy.' *SciELO 30*, 1–18. Accessed on 21 September 2022 at https://doi.org/10.1590/2526-8910.ctoRE252733032

Young, S. (2014) 'I'm not your inspiration, thank you very much.' TEDx Talk, June. Accessed on 1 October 2022 at www.ted.com/talks/stella_young_i_m_not_your_inspiration_thank_you_very_much/transcript?language=en

CHAPTER THREE

Typical Teenage Years Plus Cerebral Palsy

I wish I knew then what I know now as the disruptor in me wouldn't have let that one go by so easily.

From the start, my education was compromised due to systemic ableism and microaggressions; my parents had to fight very hard to create an accessible environment where I could thrive. In primary school I wasn't as aware of the implications of systemic ableism in the educational system and the repercussions of this on my school experience. I still went to school and played with my friends, which was all that I cared about. However, when I reached secondary school this all changed, and I became increasingly aware of the injustices happening around me.

In occupational science, the study of occupational therapy, humans are viewed as occupational beings as we have the desire to use our time in a purposeful way. This desire comes from health and survival needs, which are influenced by socio-cultural forces. Therefore, as a result of these needs not being met, engagement in occupations becomes an innate desire, enabling us to 'flourish' (Wilcox 1993). But if occupations are so integral to our humans needs, then of course transitioning between occupations is going to have a repercussion on each aspect of an individual's life. Occupational transitions are changes such as starting school, entering puberty, moving through education and getting a job (Lim and Jones 2017). Transitioning from primary to secondary school is a big enough change for anyone, never mind adding a disability, and thus more societal barriers, to the mix.

My transition to secondary school was obviously complicated, but we had a process that worked – my parents and I had been on multiple visits during the two years prior to me moving schools. We worked with my physiotherapist and occupational therapist to ensure that everything was put into place. I'd been attending Transition Club and everything felt right. I was enjoying this element of early planning (Lim and Jones 2017) as it enabled me to work out ways I could enjoy my experience as a disabled student. However, I didn't want to leave my one-to-one support from primary school behind, and I remember begging her to come to secondary school with me ('I don't think it quite works like that, Georgia'). The transition to a new support system was hard. There were a lot of environmental changes such as different classes and different teachers, as well as adjusting to different expectations, which, as you can imagine, was quite demanding for my disabled 12-year-old self. Beyond academic changes, there was a significant difference in the way that lessons were taught and delivered. Primary school had a nurturing aspect while secondary school was more focused on students' academic achievements, so this was another element of change. And outside of the classroom, there was an increased focus on homework (Lim and Jones 2017), which added a new dimension to the way I managed my disability.

It was, for obvious reasons, very important to me that my one-to-one support always took the time to get to know me. I'll be honest, I wasn't the biggest fan of having to build a relationship with multiple teaching assistants for each school subject. I did enjoy getting to know these lovely people, but it took time to get to know how I worked. I had a lot of internalized ableism and worried that I might get judged or that the teaching assistants might not like the way I worked. After having consistent one-to-one support in primary school, working with new teaching assistants in different subjects was an adjustment. On the other hand, I didn't need support in every subject, and I soon enjoyed having that mix of support and independent work.

There were a few initial problems. For example, I once got disciplined for pulling an energy drink out of my bag when it was in my EHCP that I needed this to help with energy levels! This happened quite often in school with supply teachers who didn't believe that having an energy drink was part of my access requirements. In this particular situation, I needed this energy boost as I was feeling drained from having my vaccinations, not that I should have had to justify that! It's fair to say that my parents and learning mentor weren't impressed with the supply teacher's handling of this situation. Looking back, it would have really helped me if I had carried with me physical proof to showcase my medical exemptions. I remember crying – not because I had been given detention, but because I was angry about their ableist attitude. A supply teacher who had no prior knowledge of me or my disability had not believed me and made me justify my access requirements in front of the whole class – I was fuming! Being disciplined was out of my normal behavioural pattern as I was once inclined to be a goody two-shoes; not that you'd believe that now, as I'm a proud rebellious disruptor! My upset that day was more due to the fact of it being a ridiculous reason for discipline for which I had to publicly justify my medical needs; it was both wrong and ableist!

Despite this happening over a decade ago, I wanted to include it here because reflecting on my life and writing this book has made me realize how much ableism I did face, and how much of this I've internalized. I remember my parents being so angry about this situation and I didn't really understand why. It's not just about the supply teacher, however; it's about the everyday assumptions and prejudices that I, and the disabled community, face because we live our lives a bit differently.

Anyway, back to the point. Year 7 had a lot of changes, another one being that I only saw my close friends from primary school at lunch and break times because they weren't in my half of the year. Being the chatterbox I am, I soon befriended new classmates and got into a new routine, although this was another new element to contend with alongside everything else...all this mixed in with chronic fatigue was exhausting!

The reason that I was in the other half of the year to my close friends was that I was placed in one of the 'lower sets', which, of course, did my self-esteem wonders. In all honesty, I knew I wasn't the brightest of the bunch – yes, I know, insert internalized ableism here. I was aware that I didn't get the highest SATs score, and to my 12-year-old-self it felt right to be placed in one of the lower sets. Standardized Assessments Tests (SATs) are taken in primary school – these test scores that you get in the last year of primary school are used to determine your ability and the sets you are placed into at secondary school. Therefore, when I was approached at the end of Year 7 and told that I would be moving up into a higher set, I was thrilled!

The move took some time, and it wasn't until the December of Year 8 that I made the transition to the new set. As excited as I was, mainly to be in a few classes with my close friends of course, I was really nervous during this process. What if I couldn't keep up with my peers? My internalized ableism made me question if school had made the right decision, if I would belong in those classes – not to mention that I had to make new friends again within a new class. Not going to lie, I did make some pretty embarrassing moves to try and make friends, but moving classes honestly made me feel like the new girl (who was also wobbly, dribbled a lot, and nine times out of ten had her lunch spilled down her uniform) – it was tough!

Like I say, I've never thought of myself as academic, and internalized ableism was heavily weighing down on me in terms of 'fitting in'. Even having support from the teaching assistants was a different dynamic to how it had been in the previous set.

Changing my classes resulted in being placed in the very top set in technology and I was so adamant I didn't belong there because I 'wasn't intelligent enough'. Writing these words now feels so ridiculous; I was doing woodwork and my intelligence level didn't matter as my fine motor needs meant I always needed support anyway! Yet I felt the need to prove I belonged there and I worked so hard to do so. My hard work was recognized and it benefited me through being moved up to higher sets again within some subjects. But the feeling of belonging, which is fundamental for human motivation (Maslow 1943), was still not there.

Remember that I still didn't know what ableism or internalized ableism was at this stage of my life, but a year or so after moving up, this overwhelming feeling of not belonging all made sense. At Parents' Evening a year later, it was suggested that I was where I was always meant to be, and that I never should have been *judged based on my disability*. My parents and I had almost figured this out for ourselves, but to hear the words come out of a teacher's mouth was unbelievable; I just couldn't believe how blunt they were about the discrimination I'd suffered! I felt this also put the onus on me due to having a disability, and that it was my 'fault', making me feel like a burden. I felt stereotyped as the *young*, *'vulnerable'*, *disabled girl* and that I needed more support due to this. I never should have had to feel like this; I could still be in a higher set and need support, yet I felt that not enough thought was given to my actual access needs. I predominantly needed physical support rather than support towards my intellectual learning. For example, in maths I eventually ended up in the top set. I received one-to-one support with maths teachers in this set as they could easily understand the mathematical terminology. I needed transcription, not support because I didn't understand maths.

I understand my academic privileges, but the question here is, are we critically looking at systems, or are we just stereotyping and putting people into boxes? My sister once saw a chart that showed herself as one of the students who had improved most across the school. Since this also included students in my school year, I asked if I was on that list, knowing I'd moved up quite a lot. When she replied 'no', it stumped me for years, but now I understand it. I hadn't improved dramatically at all; I was just eventually placed where I was always meant to be. It took so long for me to be placed there because my journey was riddled with microaggressions. I deserved better. Young people with disabilities deserve better. I wish I knew then what I know now, as the disruptor in me wouldn't have let that one go by so easily.

Yes, this book focuses on healthcare, but ableism is a wider societal and political issue. To be non-ableist, every micro, meso and macro level needs critically exploring because what's happening in school affects the whole integrated care system. If we isolated and eradicated ableism within paediatric clinics, yet it still existed in the schooling system, then the integrated care system would still be flawed and built on ableism, and it would eventually impact the paediatric clinic. To act as true allies, we must acknowledge this bigger picture and not act as bystanders just because we work in a different building or department to others.

Professional research suggests that cultural and economic criteria influence getting a diagnosis, an EHCP and entry into the right educational setting, and middle-class parents have more access to readily available support (Holt, Bowlby and Lea 2019). As a result, disabled students are more likely to be discriminated against in the classroom (due to the cost of living with a disability) and thus in peer relationships as this stigma becomes conscious (Chatzitheochari and Butler-Rees 2022). Therefore, intersectionality must be considered in order for young people to not just reach their full potential in education but also to gain a sense of belongingness. Reflecting on my teenage years as someone who comes from a working-class family, this intersectional discrimination all makes sense. I can see why I suddenly felt like I was in a different world and, with hindsight, I can see that my internalized stigma was the source of much of my own school-based drama (Chatzitheochari and Butler-Rees 2022).

When I got moved up, I went from someone who just went along with school and the academic work to someone who felt the need to 'blow their own trumpet' in everything they did. This is because of how deeply rooted my internalized ableism was at school. No matter what I achieved, I still thought my peers just saw me as the girl in the wheelchair who looked bedraggled, often having her lunch down her uniform! Yes, as I got older I could have changed my uniform at dinner to benefit my own self-esteem, but changing a shirt and tie would have been wasting spoons that I needed to get me through the afternoon.[1]

I know that I still 'blow my own trumpet' even to this day; this goes much deeper than proving that I'm more than the bedraggled, disabled girl at school who made embarrassing moves to try and make friends. Interestingly, my main group of current best friends originated from my school days, and this started because I used to sit with one of my best friends, Sophie, in art at the end of the day. Art, at the end of the day? Sophie couldn't have seen me in more of a mess if she had wanted to, and yet over ten years later we still meet up regularly.

So why did I care? I often wonder, if it wasn't for my disability, would I be so loud and feel the need to shout from the rooftops when I have something new and career-related going on? It's my job as a disabled activist to show society what disability really means. I do not post loudly about career-related milestones to be seen as an 'inspiration' because I am not. I post because, yes, I'm proud of myself, and I want to show society that my disabled life isn't that different to a non-disabled person's. I certainly know that there is a part of me that wants that validation; that's human nature. But I also want to show the world that my life with cerebral palsy is far from terrible and should not be pitied. We all have achievements that mean different things to different people, no matter who we are. The journey to get there as a disabled person may be a bit different and take a whole load more spoons, but we all have different journeys regardless of who we are.

Typical teenage drama certainly amplifies things to start with, and I found myself right in the thick of it as soon as I hit my teenage years. Beyond this, hormonal changes within myself and other students

---

1   The spoon theory is used in the chronically ill community by Christine Miserandino. It is a simple way of the community explaining how they have to save energy, and how they use more energy than others: https://butyoudontlooksick.com/articles/written-by-christine/the-spoon-theory

further complicated things (Lim and Jones 2017). During the first few years of secondary school, I was quite content with going to 'safe haven' spaces at lunchtime, not really getting involved with my peers outside of class; this worked for me during that time. I wasn't without friends, though, and I took a friend to the safe haven group most days. Yet prior to secondary school I'd never isolated myself from my peers before and I'd always had multiple friends, so why did I disengage at secondary school?

I disengaged because, as we became teenagers, the most popular thing to do was to go ice-skating on a Friday night. This just isn't accessible for me. Yes, I could have gone onto the ice in my wheelchair, but honestly, it is so boring and cold in the wheelchair on the ice rink so it was a 'no' from me. Physical environmental changes were very hard for me when some after-school and outside activities were not fully accessible for my mobility aids or my movement (Lim and Jones 2017). What I wasn't expecting was how this affected the dynamic at school. I suddenly went from having multiple friends and not needing the safe haven space to being so dependent on it that during break time I just sat outside my next class because the safe haven group didn't run then.

I really struggled with transitioning from one friendship group to another, which Lim and Jones (2017) suggest is a pattern with disabled students, and particularly those with communication impairments like myself. This period didn't last long as I was determined to make friends and not spend my last two years of secondary school like this, but I'd never had this before; I'd always had loads of friends. Don't get me wrong, it wasn't that I felt massively disliked or avoided, but some of the groups I did go to hang out with during break times didn't make me feel fully included. I'm not denying that self-loathing didn't amplify this either, but hormonal changes meant it was harder to manage situations that I had previously found easier to deal with.

All that changed when I met Sophie; Sophie was also friends with Bethany, Libby and a larger social group that I started to spend lunchtime with. Of course we were teenagers and there was still drama. The main thing is that I became close with Sophie, Bethany and Libby, and they are still my dear friends today. I couldn't believe it when we all first went out for a meal and they weren't fazed about cutting up my food. Previously, I'd internalized worries that I would become a burden if I asked friends to help me with this so I could dine out with them. In reality, I am not a burden as we all have access needs, and needing my food cut up is just one of mine!

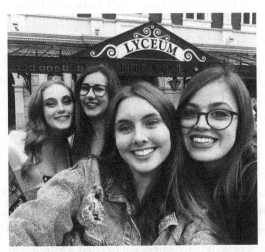

Image 3.1. *Four white females stood in front of the Lyceum Theatre. Bethany and Sophie are at the front and Libby and Georgia are behind and slightly to the left. They are smiling at the camera.*

I know I didn't get bullied at school and my experiences with friends overall wasn't bad, yet I still cried myself to sleep some nights. If this is how it made a fairly confident disabled teenager feel, then what about those who aren't? This needs to be considered by the integrated care system. The safe haven was good and I do look back on the time quite fondly, but I wanted to make friends outside of this group and carry these friendships outside of school. We all have teenage rough patches but I didn't feel supported in the transition between friendship groups as the school relied heavily on the provision of the safe haven space. Yet again, where's the person-centred practice?

Every point I've addressed so far in this chapter poses the question of whether society expects less from disabled children. It was assumed I was to be in the lower sets, and it certainly felt that school expected me to sit in the safe haven lunch club for five years. The safe haven club was really helpful, but I felt there wasn't enough recognition of the fact that I might have wanted to have or make other friends too.

Yet again this expectation comes from how society perceives disability and the fact that I was expected to live my life in a certain way and should just accept the status quo. Disabled people have opinions, wants and desires like all humans, so please don't alienate us! This alienation was often not deliberate but stemmed from the fact that the school system and teachers themselves didn't have a full understanding of disability (Lim and Jones 2017).

Sometimes I'd make the most of certain situations because I knew it would benefit me in the long term, but other times there was no chance that I was happy to accept my treatment as a disabled student. For example, at 13 I started my menstrual cycle and, just like anyone, this complex occupation was a difficult adaptation to make. Your hormones are everywhere, you're in pain, and now you have to learn how to use sanitary products. We'd had a session in school on using sanitary products, and I already knew that a sanitary towel was going to be the easiest product for me. Yet when I started my periods, which were quite heavy, I soon realized that I couldn't place the sanitary towel properly in my pants without my mum helping me. I was okay with this while everything was new, but we knew we needed a long-term solution. So mum contacted the physiotherapist to ask for support, whose advice was to use nappies.

There wasn't even a discussion when mum came off the phone, as wearing nappies was out of the question. I'd not been in nappies since I was three years old, and I was not about to start wearing them for school as a teenager. Where's the consideration of my pride and dignity? I felt that no thought was given again to me and my feelings since this was blanket advice given to everyone, so my personal circumstances weren't considered. If there was another choice, I very much doubt that any 13-year-old would want to go back to wearing nappies. Such a general 'one size fits all' approach is ableist because again it assumes that disabled people don't have thoughts, feelings and preferences but instead we would be happy to do whatever works. Well this isn't the case, and I didn't want this social exclusion or embarrassment, since getting my lunch down my uniform was enough to deal with!

In the end, my sister Matilda came up with the genius solution of mum putting the sanitary towels in my pants and me just changing my pants at school. It did take me a while to do this in the bathroom, and my close friends who knew the situation could figure out when I was on my period because I'd disappear for a while throughout the day. It was a lot better than the alternative, though.

Another example is how inter-able or disabled sex was never

discussed in sex education. I never realized at the time, but very little of what was discussed within sex education was applicable to my body – even into my twenties, I can have moments of being prudish. No one ever talked to me about sexual health in relation to my disability, and my parents didn't understand how little I knew about my own disabled body. This information should have come from healthcare professionals and be considered within the National Curriculum.

Sex is a meaningful occupation, and of course disabled people have sex – why wouldn't we? We have a libido! So why, in the 21st century, is this still a taboo subject? I know some incredible occupational therapists are doing very important work out there to raise the profile of sex as a meaningful occupation and to promote inclusive sex education, but this needs to happen earlier on. When I was old enough, an occupational therapist should have spoken to me about this. I may have been embarrassed as a teenager, but I'd rather be embarrassed than have the school's ableist lack of relatable sex education. Again, I know I'm talking about something that happened over a decade ago, and I was thrilled to see sexuality and intimacy being addressed at the Royal College of Occupational Therapists, Children, Young People and Families Specialist Section Conference in 2022 (Schmidt 2022), but these conversations are still not being normalized into mainstream health and sex education, and there's still so much work to do to challenge perceptions and established norms in order to give disabled people the rights they deserve.

Between being put in the wrong sets, teenage drama and having to go along with an ableist National Curriculum, it's fair to say my teenage years weren't an easy ride. But it wasn't just me whose teenage years were altered because of my disability, since this affected my whole family, including my sister. My sister, **Matilda Vine**, had more ableist experiences than I did at school, all because she was known as 'Georgia Vine's sister'. How is this fair? Matilda is her own person and she needed to live her own life. As children, Matilda and I certainly had a different relationship than most siblings. We did everything together, so much so that we often got mistaken for twins. Obviously, I loved being so close and I'm thankful for this, but sometimes we had to attend events as a pair because of my needs and how our life worked. We both had a great childhood, but I do realize that Matilda compromised a lot because my needs required more support from our parents.

Going to secondary school should have been her time to shine and show the world what Matilda Vine is capable of. She did do this, and I'm immensely proud of what she achieved, yet knowing she was predominantly known as 'Georgia Vine's sister' did not sit well with me. She's her own wonderful, intelligent self and she should be recognized for this. I interviewed Matilda about her experiences growing up on my blog in 2021, and she said that 'I often felt lonely or unappreciated growing up as the attention failed to remain on me.' I come from a working-class family where my parents did their best to manage work, life and the responsibilities of having a disabled child, but the implications of this probably still weigh heavily on Matilda to this day. Holistic practice needs to be considered for families, and I know Matilda felt this having interviewed her for previous work I've done. Why aren't there more support networks for siblings? How can we give non-disabled siblings the occupational justice they deserve?

'An insight into being the non-disabled sibling: An interview with my sister' captures **Matilda**'s experiences, and gives us more food for thought on this area of practice (Vine 2021).

A report from Hastings (2014), who worked with the charity Sibs,[2] found that siblings of disabled children are more at risk for psychological and social complexities. However, there is limited research on this area, so more work needs to be done as we cannot be anti-ableist without looking at the bigger picture. In my story, my sister's experiences played a massive part of this and should not be ignored.

Sibs is a UK charity that represents both adults and children who have disabled siblings as well as offering advice for parents and professionals.

---

2   www.sibs.org.uk/about-sibs

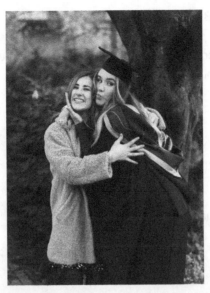

Image 3.2. *Two white females. Matilda, on the right, is pouting and looking off to the side, wearing a cap and gown for her graduation. Her arms are around her sister Georgia, who is in a fluffy coat; Georgia is smiling. There is a tree behind them.*

When re-reading this chapter, I'm questioning what I've written because I'm not looking for a sympathy card. I did have some lovely experiences at secondary school and during my early teenage years, although it's fair to say that I experienced quite a lot of ableism without even realizing, and accepted inequalities too often because I thought that was just the way that life was. Now it is evident to me that the integrated care system during these years wasn't what it should have been, even with an EHCP in place. Imagine how hard it must be for those families who don't have a diagnosis or EHCP, both of which provide access and support to enable their child to reach their full potential. If we want to become successful allies, we all need to start including disabled people and their families to ensure that their healthcare and education is equal.

NOT SO TERRIBLE...P.A.L.S.Y. REFLECTIVE LOG
Pausing
Stop and think about what you have read in this chapter. What are your main takeaway points? What are your main questions?

. . . .

. . . .

. . . .

Analysing
Why did this resonate with you?

. . . .

. . . .

. . . .

Learning
What did you learn from this?

. . . .

. . . .

. . . .

Solving
What actions need to be put into place?

. . . .

. . . .

. . . .

Your plan
How will you achieve these actions? What are your goals?

. . . .

. . . .

. . . .

References

Chatzitheochari, S. and Butler-Rees, A. (2022) 'Disability, social class and stigma: An intersectional analysis of disabled young people's school experiences.' *Sociology.* Accessed on 2 December 2022 at https://doi.org/10.1177/00380385221133710

Hastings, R. (2014) 'Children and adolescents who are the siblings of children with intellectual disability or autism: Research evidence.' Sibs, University of Warwick. Accessed on 15 January 2022 at www.sibs.org.uk/supporting-young-siblings/professionals/needs-of-young-siblings/children-and-adolescents-who-are-the-siblings-of-children-with-intellectual-disabilities-or-autism-research-evidence-professor-richard-hasting-2013

Holt, L., Bowlby, S. and Lea, J. (2019) 'Disability, special educational needs, class, capitals and segregation in schools: A population geography perspective.' *Population, Space and Place* 25, 4, 1–11. Accessed on 2 December 2022 at https://doi.org/10.1002/psp.2229

Lim, S.M. and Jones, F. (2017) 'Occupational Transitions for Children and Young People.' In S. Rodger and A. Kennedy-Behr (eds) *Occupation-Centred Practice with Children: A Practical Guide for Occupational Therapists* (Chapter 6). Chichester: John Wiley & Sons Ltd.

Maslow, A.H. (1943) 'A theory of human motivation.' *Psychological Review* 50, 4, 370–396.

Schmidt, E. (2022) 'Promoting Occupational Equity and Justice by Addressing Sexuality and Intimacy among Youth with Disabilities.' Paper Presentation. Royal College of Occupational Therapists, Children, Young People and Families Conference, 11 November.

Vine, G. (2021) 'An insight into being the non-disabled sibling: An interview with my sister.' *Not So Terrible Palsy* [Blog], 24 September. Accessed on 15 January 2023 at https://notsoterriblepalsy.com/2021/09/24/an-insight-into-being-the-non-disabled-sibling-an-interview-with-my-sister

Wilcox, A. (1993) 'A theory of the human need for occupation.' *Journal of Occupational Science* 1, 1, 17–24. Accessed on 14 January 2023 at https://doi.org/10.1080/14427591.1993.9686375

CHAPTER FOUR

The Sudden Stop in Services

Not only was it fraught when I transitioned to sixth form; it just felt a million miles away from the reality that I'd been used to.

I was 17 when I started to get involved in disabled activism. Naturally I had questions as my interpretation of the world around me had now been enhanced. I'd always taken every societal and systemic barrier I faced with a pinch of salt with the typical teenager view of saying 'Mum/Dad, don't!' whenever they wanted to question or complain about something (although they were always right). Yet I now know what really fuelled my activism was my lack of support during my transition into adulthood, and this is when I started to not just passively let the noise happen, but to make the noise myself.

The transition into adulthood can be the most significant across a person's lifespan due to negotiating the different pathways and life experiences (Lim and Jones 2017). My experiences of disability and all the corresponding red tape throughout the first 16 years of my life had certainly amplified my anxiety about this. I even remember being more cautious about the options I picked to study for my GCSEs (General Certificate of Secondary Education) in terms of my future career. Had I known then what I know now, I would have certainly worried less, yet every decision with a disability has so much more complexity and consequences.

However, my transition from children's services wasn't the planned process that I was longing for. When I was discharged I felt abandoned. Now you'd think that I'd enjoy not having to attend appointments all the time, giving me more time to be a typical 17-year-old, but in all honesty, I was petrified. Any disability-related query, qualm or worry I had throughout my life had been sorted out by the paediatric multidisciplinary team on the other end of the phone. And I often found that when the team couldn't actually answer my query themselves, they always knew where to direct me. Yet overnight, this support network had disappeared, and I felt quite alone.

Not only did I feel alone, so did my parents. So before we analyse this, let's get some thoughts from their perspective...

How did you feel when I was discharged from children's services?
Mum: Disgusted, there was no support whatsoever. There was no help regarding your next steps. They asked me if it was okay for them to close your case and I said no because you still needed the consultant to write reports to enable you to get the support you needed for university.

You needed it then more than ever to enable your transition to adulthood and give guidance towards your next steps. Your needs had not changed, so why would you no longer need support? Why do your needs change at 16? Yes, you're more mature, but you still needed guidance; we also needed guidance as a family unit. This stage is complicated for anyone without adding a disability into the mix.

I phoned the service to ask for signposting and was given nothing; I was told that there wasn't anything out there. There was not even an integrated care system to help you transition to college. I couldn't believe that that was it; I became alone overnight.

Dad: I feel that the transition into adulthood was fraught and filled with disappointment and disbelief. After fighting for support throughout your schooling, we found that most, if not all, support ended upon completion of secondary education. I felt disappointed with the system and found it lacking in empathy towards what should be an important step in any teenager's life, regardless of their ability.

Why was that?
Mum: There should be support available for every transition you're going through, so I felt massively let down when I'd put in all the effort as a parent and they couldn't offer me anything. I'd always had someone to go to for advice and support, and now there was

nothing, which weighed heavily on me mentally; I couldn't sleep because of the worry. We were left to navigate an ableist society by ourselves; we were petrified and wracked with anticipation for what would come next.

[Just want to note that I may have helped with getting some phrases down on paper in this answer; I think you can guess which one... hehehe!]

Dad: As a parent, I felt the loss of support affected our lives massively. The reliance on healthcare professionals stopped overnight and this left us in a world without anyone to turn to. This affected my mental health and caused stress and strain throughout the family, so it was a dark period of our lives.

How could this be better?

Mum: Not only weren't your current needs considered, neither were your future education and career. More support was needed in all areas such as signposting and more discussions about your future, but there was nothing. The process also needed to be more gradual rather than just ending in the abrupt way that it did.

We needed more support with everything, such as how you were going to get to college and back and transitioning to university; we felt in the dark and needed someone there for us. Luckily you went to a very supportive college who helped us a lot. Without the support from college, we would have been lost. For example, they directed us to a source we didn't know about where we could get funding regarding transport to college.

The availability of support for us wasn't there to accommodate our circumstances. Support groups were available but again, didn't fit in with busy family life. Not to mention how hard it was to manage the exhaustion of this turmoil. Why is this education around transitions not delivered as part of an integrated care package? The jigsaw puzzle is not finished and the bigger picture needs to be considered.

Dad: An integrated health, education and welfare system would have helped. There should have been more education available to us and more programmed information for every transition. Again, we were left to find out the information ourselves and I felt that the system was built on ableist assumptions, meaning that financial support was very limited and not easy to source. Luckily your college helped as much as they could to provide us with sources of information to help your experience at sixth form.

What advice would you give to other parents just starting out on this journey?

Mum: My advice would be to be realistic about what works for individual families to be able to function. Don't give up and carry on; there is information out there, even if you have to source it yourself, which I hope is easier to find now than it was for us.

This needs to be more accessible, however – what if you haven't got the money to aid this research and haven't got the support network to help?

I hope my personal honest opinion has helped. This was a hard time of our lives; every transition is difficult, and I hope that more education is given to make people aware of their entitlements.

This worry never goes away. I worry about the future and consider what this may look like as we age as well. More compassion and understanding is needed to increase the awareness of just how much work and planning goes into daily life. Who knows what the future holds? We will continue to work together to navigate this, and hope that one day we will receive better support from allies.

Dad: I would reiterate everything that your mum has said. Don't give up. I hope research is available at your fingertips; join forums, network and speak to as many other parents/carers who will readily give advice and information as you can. Don't feel you're alone as there are thousands of helpful people willing to give support and information in order to help you in most situations. In my experience, the more effort you put in, the greater the outcome.

What key things should professionals know to be able to support other families like ours?

Mum: In the future, I would hope for professionals to look at people as individuals as well as working with the family to establish realistic goals. Furthermore, it's important to support individuals to navigate their future and reach their full potential rather than being so focused on developmental milestones from the start.

Dad: There should be someone who can talk you through this transition and also highlight future areas of your life where you would need more support, for example how to make a claim for financial support. In any other areas of life, you would have professional help to fill out forms such as pensions, mortgages and buying a car. But when it comes to accessing financial, medical and support at work, there are so many additional anxieties. Don't be afraid to push and be your family's primary advocate.

Firstly, I'd like to thank both of my parents for all their contributions. I know all the interviews were tough, and this last interview was by far the hardest, as frankly this is still a sensitive topic. The most crucial thing that I want to unpack is the lack of support. At a time when our family unit needed support the most due to changes in the expectations and demands in my occupational performance (Lim and Jones 2017), it wasn't there. As my parents concluded, this lack of support at a time of change and need caused more stress. This was particularly important when thinking about my future.

Lim and Jones (2017) state that in order for transition to be successful, especially for those whose options are limited in society, they need to pass GCSE maths and English. I acknowledge my privileges academically, yet honestly, stating that individuals are required to attain certain grades to be able to access most roles in society – can you get any more ableist? Disability, social class and ethnicity have a significant impact on differentials in educational attainment in both primary and secondary schools, meaning that we must consider the multitude of societal barriers that young disabled people face (Chatzitheochari and Platt 2018), and the profound, long-lasting effect that this has on their transition into adulthood. These barriers are exacerbated if the young disabled person and their family do not have access to a reliable support system, research or signposting on their conditions and funding towards support. I acknowledge my privilege that, despite coming from a working-class family, my parents had the time to research funding methods to aid my transition and support my learning journey.

Chatzitheochari and Platt's (2018) research found that university expectations had a strong effect on educational transitions, resulting in the stigma around this being internalized. It is also important to note that this is largely dependent on parental expectations. My parents never pushed me to do anything I didn't want to, and just wanted me to thrive as any supportive parent would. I think the reason why I felt more pressure academically is because I knew I had to face more societal barriers. I would have done anything I could to make this easier and to allow myself more options for the future.

The increase in pressure, anxiety and need for more support was already building before we began transitioning, never mind during the transition. Ryan *et al.* (2022) suggest that more time is needed for the transition period so it can be carefully planned and reflected on by the whole multidisciplinary team. In reality, the transition often feels rushed, and our family certainly felt abandoned and lost as there was little consideration of my future needs and transitions. Even my support to go to college was minimal; like my mum pointed out, if my college hadn't been as supportive, we could have easily found ourselves becoming more lost. I found it very insightful to read Lim and Jones (2017) when they described the transition from secondary school to further education as 'fraught with challenges'; *fraught* was the exact same word that my dad used to describe this period.

Not only was it fraught when I transitioned to sixth form; it just felt a million miles away from the reality that I'd been used to. For example, during my first year of college, I embarked on a trip abroad to Berlin. I remember ticking the 'maybe' box when we provisionally registered our interest in the trip. Hats off to my parents who were more brave than me on this one, and said I should change my answer to 'yes'. Registering an interest was the easy part, yet the disability-related planning wasn't as intense as I'd expected in the five months that followed. I remember being in a planning meeting alongside my parents and a college teacher, thinking, where is the input from a healthcare professional?

I had the best five days of my life in Berlin; it gave me the boost I needed into helping me become more of my own person and getting the sense of my new reality with no input from healthcare professionals. College were really supportive too, and didn't hold me back from doing anything that I felt that I could manage during the trip. Yet planning this did affect me mentally.

When I had attended a five-day residential trip less than an hour away from home in Year 6, I had endured months of planning with healthcare professionals who concluded I could only manage four days. Yet going abroad – nothing. Given, I was a lot older and had more autonomy and understanding of my disability, but it felt a big change to go from being over-cautious to what now felt like being totally under-prepared. It was hard for both my parents and me to accept. Yes, we understood my needs, but everything we had done prior to me starting college needed careful consideration and a stamp of approval from my consultant, occupational therapist and physiotherapist. So not needing to jump through these rigorous hoops felt nerve-wracking and, to use my dad's word again...fraught!

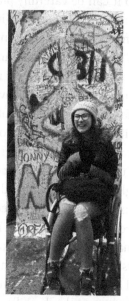

Image 4.1. *Georgia, a white female, aged 17, in her manual wheelchair. She has glasses and a woolly hat on. She is laughing and is seated in front of part of the Berlin Wall.*

It's not just my parents and I who felt this confusion. Ryan *et al.* (2022) found that young people with cerebral palsy across the UK report similar experiences. They highlight the lack of transparency with some individuals not knowing if they'd even been referred to adult services. I knew that I had not been referred to adult services and had experienced little signposting. I was told that if I felt I needed any support again, that I would have to go to the GP and get a referral to adult services. According to Ryan *et al.* (2022), many families were unaware if their GP even knew that they had been discharged from children's services. We certainly weren't sure if our GP understood that I had been discharged, so this amplified our worries. It also reinforced my internalized ableism as I was then made to feel like I shouldn't require the support. I've been discharged from children's services for over half a decade now, and I've only recently asked for a physiotherapy referral for my CP muscular-related pain levels. Only recently have I been able to give myself validation for needing that support, and this is only as a result of talking to others with similar experiences.

Colver *et al.* (2018) highlight the need to give young people more confidence to manage their condition and develop health self-advocacy skills. As an individual who has experienced the transition from using children's services to using 'adult services', I couldn't agree with this more; it has taken me many years to accept that it is okay that my health is changing and that I need more support. This confidence has only come with age and my experiences as an occupational therapist and disabled activist. My 17-year-old self would have gained a lot from being taught these essential health self-advocacy skills. Not only does this enable me to have better autonomy over my health, but it also validates my feelings, and would certainly have reduced the internalized ableism I felt around 'exaggerating my disability' in my late teens.

As I said, I only went to the GP about a physiotherapy referral after talking to my friends **Chloe Tear**[1] and **Ellie Simpson**, who I met through online forums. Chloe is an award-winning disability blogger and freelance writer and Ellie is the founder of the charity CP Teens UK.[2] CP Teens UK has had a massive impact on me in enabling me to be more confident as a young disabled woman. I never hated being disabled but, after my teenage years, my ability to live my disabled life confidently had reduced. Meeting others such as Chloe and Ellie helped me to realize how much I love being disabled and what an utter joy it is to be a part of the disabled community. I have had many wonderful adventures with my fellow 'wobbly amigos', and I cannot wait for more!

As thankful as I am to have made wonderful friends, I do wonder if my self-advocacy would be different now if I had not fully immersed myself in the disabled community the way I did during my late teens.

---

1   https://chloetear.co.uk
2   www.cpteensuk.org

This is why good communication is essential within the integrated care system during the transition from children's services to adult services, to ensure that a beneficial transition plan is made (Lim and Jones 2017). Again, this is a process that must include the individual (Colver *et al.* 2018) as well as everyone involved in the journey rather than the plan just being devised by professionals and handed to the individual, like my transition plan was.

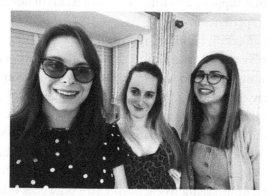

Image 4.2. Three white females. Chloe is on the left, wearing tinted glasses and a polka-dot top. Ellie is in the middle, wearing leopard print, and Georgia is on the end, with her glasses on, wearing a cropped top and cardigan.

Lim and Jones (2017) state that transition plans include goals targeted for those with learning disabilities, and mine certainly felt like this. As I have no lived experience of a learning disability, I can't comment on the suitability of these transition plans for those who do, but for me personally, they weren't suitable. My transition plan included things such as what I like to do in my spare time and who I live with. This was a document that I was advised to take with me to job interviews, yet it was irrelevant as I could easily have told the interviewers the facts that it covered. Again, I'm not denying that this format may work for those with other access needs, but for me, it wasn't suitable. I'd personally much rather my potential employer got to know me over time rather than reading from a piece of paper. I acknowledge my biases, but this is much bigger than young adults with cerebral palsy. Less than a third of autistic people have enough time to prepare for transition into adulthood (All-Party Parliamentary Group on Autism 2019), so we need to look at this systemically to develop specific services, using universal strategies that address the needs of adolescents going through this huge and complex transition (Ryan *et al.* 2022). This will enhance equitability across all children's services.

Colver *et al.* (2018) looked into transition coordinators and found that, although they could help, their role wasn't useful, as longer-term relationships were needed to develop trust and confidence. My last appointment under children's services was with an occupational therapist I didn't know, meaning that I didn't receive any closure. I needed someone who knew my long-term needs and understood me holistically. I feel that's also why my transition plan felt confusing and undermining. I was made to feel as though I didn't understand my own needs, which did not sit well with me as someone who was going on to study the same profession a year later.

I'm aware that systemic changes can't be made overnight, and I know that paediatric occupational therapists do know about the flaws within this area of practice. The majority of the time when I've been asked to give a talk or guest lecture about my experiences, it has been about my transition into adulthood, as many know that big systemic changes need to be made. There are a few hurdles that can be removed, and we can do this through solutions such as providing an education package, as my mum suggested.

We, as a family, felt like we were navigating a society built on systemic ableism alone, and we know that this gap cannot be solely pinpointed to one area. However, some kind of educational package would have been useful to help this new reality seem less scary. This transition is not just about choosing the right career path; even now, in my twenties, I still haven't got everything prepared to live my life the way I want to. Although I stopped putting time frames on goals a long time ago as I don't think life quite works like that, even without the extra complications of a disability, it would have been useful to look at my life stages from a holistic perspective, because we needed some consideration of my future access needs. Yes, of course I'm going to need physiotherapy in the future again, and self-managing this is going to be different, but I can adapt to this throughout adulthood. But I now need support in other areas of my life.

Truth be told, as I write this I'm at a bit of a loss as I am hoping that I will soon be able to move out of the family home. I know that putting everything into place for this won't be easy and will certainly be a long process. This includes an accessible home, sourcing a PA (personal assistant) and learning new skills, such as cooking, in an adaptive way. Occupational transitions such as moving out are already complex, big life steps, and adding the challenges of a chronic health condition does complicate this even further, leaving me feeling lost.

Moving out as a disabled adult has additional challenges, and solving this takes up so much more energy. Staying at home for a longer period than I originally anticipated has been beneficial, as otherwise I wouldn't have been able to invest in my career while planning on moving out. I've accepted this and I don't necessarily have a date in mind as I shouldn't let societal norms determine my life plan. My transition into adulthood is still filled with so much uncertainty. If I had a transition plan on what moving out may look like, that would enable me to have more understanding of the services I may need help from on this journey. Not only would my anxiety decrease, but I would also be more excited and motivated to start this process rather than constantly worrying about the known or unknown hurdles I may face.

TOP TIPS

✓ Plan, plan and plan – you can never plan too much with a disability to save those spoons!

✓ Don't give up – I really hope the transition process has improved since experiencing it myself, but if it hasn't, do your own research and create your own networks where possible. Charities like CP Teens UK will help along the way by providing you with a support network of those who have had similar experiences.

✓ Don't be afraid to ask for more support where you need it, whether this is from healthcare professionals, schools or peers. This is your life, so make sure you're getting as much support and information as you need!

Occupational transitions have many layers, thus placing occupational therapists in a unique position to help young people and families navigate this period. To make the change from using children's services to using adult services successful, it needs to be critically explored by more than just occupational therapists, though. We need to work on this as a collective to enhance support throughout this process in order to enable young people to thrive.

NOT SO TERRIBLE...P.A.L.S.Y. REFLECTIVE LOG

Pausing

Stop and think about what you have read in this chapter. What are your main takeaway points? What are your main questions?

....

....

....

Analysing

Why did this resonate with you?

....

....

....

Learning

What did you learn from this?

....

....

....

Solving

What actions need to be put into place?

....

....

....

Your plan

How will you achieve these actions? What are your goals?

....

....

....

References

All-Party Parliamentary Group on Autism (2019) *The Autism Act, 10 Years On: A Report from the All-Party Parliamentary Group on Autism on Understanding, Services and Support for Autistic People and Their Families in England.* The National Autistic Society.

Chatzitheochari, S. and Platt, L. (2018) 'Disability differential in educational attainment in England: Primary and secondary effects.' *The British Journal of Sociology 70*, 2, 502–525. Accessed on 13 January 2023 at https://doi.org/10.1111/1468-4446.12372

Colver, A., Pearse, R., Watson, R.M., Fay, M., Rapley, T., Mann, K.D., Le Couter, A., Parr, J.R. and McConachie, H. (2018) 'How well do services for young people with long term conditions deliver features proposed to improve transition?' *BMC Health Services Research 18*, 337. Accessed on 14 January 2023 at https://doi.org/10.1186/s12913-018-3168-9

Lim, S.M. and Jones, F. (2017) 'Occupational Transitions for Children and Young People.' In S. Rodger and A. Kennedy-Behr (eds) *Occupation-Centred Practice with Children: A Practical Guide for Occupational Therapists* (Chapter 6). Chichester: John Wiley & Sons Ltd.

Ryan, J.M., Walsh, M., Owens, M., Byrne, M., Kroll, T., Hensey, O., Kerr, C., Norris, M., Walsh, M., Lavelle, G. and Fortune, H. (2022) 'Transition to adult service experienced by young people with cerebral palsy: A cross-sectional study.' *Developmental Medicine & Child Neurology 65*, 2, 285–293. Accessed on 14 January 2023 at https://doi.org/10.1111/dmcn.15317

PART TWO

Reflecting on My Occupational Therapy Training

CHAPTER FIVE

The Lead-Up to Studying Occupational Therapy

In my personal statement, I spoke about my personal experiences of occupational therapy and how my disability is my tool, and now I've kind of made a career based on this fact!

I've always aspired to go to university from a very young age; I remember being around seven when my older cousin graduated, and I knew that I wanted to follow in her footsteps. I loved school and was very passionate about my education, which was greatly influenced by my parents, although they never pushed me to go to university. I knew that I wanted to do a degree and was involved in programmes with the University of Sheffield from the age of 14.

Deciding what I wanted to do at university wasn't straightforward. Looking back I put a lot of pressure on myself to achieve and fulfil my potential. At the age of 16 I had narrowed what I wanted to study at university down to two options: either occupational therapy or maths. I know, I know, I've heard it all before – these two subjects are polar opposites. I did always enjoy maths at school, though, finding myself skilled at the subject and fairly quick to catch on. I had fallen in love with the subject at a young age and I did not like the thought of suddenly leaving maths behind after eating, sleeping and breathing it at A-Level. Although one thing I wouldn't miss were the presumptions and ableism I faced studying maths – I've lost count of the amount of people who automatically thought I was retaking GCSE maths when I told them I was taking maths at college.

I'd also taken health and social care alongside studying psychology at college, which I had purposefully chosen with the idea of potentially wanting to study occupational therapy. They were certainly the right subjects for me, and I enjoyed psychology a great deal more than I thought I would.

So the summer of 2017 came, and it was time to make my final decision between maths and occupational therapy. It was my family who suggested that occupational therapy was probably more for me and that they felt that's where my true passion would be; looking back, they were absolutely right! Plus, I thought occupational therapy certainly has that problem-solving element to it that I knew I would miss when leaving my studies of maths behind me.

With hindsight I can, of course, look at this through a very different lens and add a whole new perspective. Problem-solving and finding the answer are two different things, and this is where occupational therapy is so different to maths as we are not 'fixing' in occupational therapy and looking for a definitive answer, but instead we are trying to adapt. There is also no 'wrong answer' in occupational therapy as different people can find different ways to participate in an occupation through completely varied routes.

During the summer I went for a driving assessment to see what adaptations I'd need to drive with my cerebral palsy. I remember telling my assessor that I was heading into my final year of college, so, of course they asked me whether I was continuing to study and what I was going to study. When I mentioned that I was choosing to study occupational therapy (after months of deliberation between that and maths!), it turned out that the assessor was an occupational therapist! This was so eye-opening as it showed me how diverse occupational therapy was and how many varied jobs there were out there, working with all age groups and individuals in so many different settings. I was once asked if I could name a setting where an occupational therapist couldn't work and I couldn't think of one – you can scope out a role for an occupational therapist anywhere!

After that summer I began to apply to university through UCAS (the Universities and Colleges Admissions Service),[1] so, of course...bring on the red tape! UCAS is the system that we apply through in the UK to the vast majority of universities. There are often different application processes if you are applying for other courses that run independently,

---

1   www.ucas.com

but the overarching idea is that this is a regulated, fair system. Each UK student is given access to an online platform where they prepare their personal statement alongside being granted numeral points for each grade they achieve during their studies. Again, I knew this wouldn't be as straightforward for me and I'd prepared myself for my UCAS application to take a little bit longer, as that's just life with a disability.

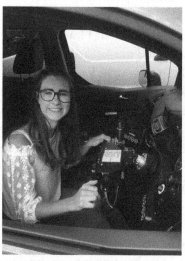

Image 5.1. *Georgia, a white female, sat in her car with her hands on a tiler (how she drives, like bike handle bars). She is wearing a white top and smiling at the camera.*

I had no idea where I was going to study at university and I'd applied to a few different places within an hour of Sheffield. Staying at home was my preferred option, but after no movement on my UCAS application, I was getting nervous! I'd applied to four occupational therapy courses and one health and human sciences course at the University of Sheffield. This was my back-up plan, as advised by the college, but my conditional offer asked for higher grades than the occupational therapy courses, so this was clearly never going to happen.

A lecturer from one university who offered me a conditional offer took me to one side during my interview and said how inaccessible the university was and advised this shouldn't be my firm choice. I wholeheartedly appreciate this honesty from the university, but my word, isn't it frustrating that inaccessibility is still so common? My dad and I soon discovered how inaccessible this environment was ourselves, and this ruled that university off our list!

TOP TIPS

✓ Always go on a campus tour on open days and don't make the mistake I made here by not having the time to fit one in, as clearly I wasted a whole lot of spoons! Campus tours are helpful to ask current students pertinent questions, but also to find out about access requirements and meeting your potential future lecturers.

✓ Always go to the open day prepared with a list of questions you'd like to ask.

The next two interviews came; they were a good experience overall, apart from the fact that back-to-back interviews are so difficult for someone with chronic fatigue, so this was not ideal! Yet weeks went by with no offers from both universities, and those weeks turned into months. This is pretty common for some courses as they are continuing to go down their lists and processing all of the students they have left to interview. But it still doesn't make this process less nerve-wracking at the age of 18!

Meanwhile I got rejected from Sheffield Hallam University. Yes, this is where I ended up studying. Meanwhile I got rejected from Sheffield Hallam University. Yes, this is where I ended up studying. Confused? Let me explain. I got a straight-up rejection, without interview, on an *interviewable* course, by someone in the admissions team at Sheffield Hallam because I didn't meet the entry grades – despite my personal tutor specifying that I was already meeting my predicted grades, and was therefore on track to get higher grades.

At the time, I just took it on the chin. I thought that it was just one of those things, and a few other of my peers had got rejections at this point, so I was not alone. But my personal tutor made me realize how wrong this was and we decided to appeal. I'm so glad I did as my appeal was accepted and I got an interview and then received a conditional offer that then got changed to unconditional after putting Sheffield Hallam as my first choice. Part of me did want to leave Sheffield and get a taste of 'university life' with independent living to build up more skills for adulthood, but I knew I wasn't ready as my disability-related anxiety was far too high. At that point, I was struggling to get a taxi by myself due to my anxiety, never mind moving out.

Looking back now, I made the right decision, and wholeheartedly believe that I wouldn't be sat here today, writing this book, if I hadn't gone to Sheffield Hallam University, as they were my biggest supporters for my blog *Not So Terrible Palsy*.

Oh, what about the other universities? I had to have additional meetings with the other two universities to see if they could *accommodate* my needs. I understand they needed to see me for this, but making my way across the country for additional meetings while trying to focus on my A-Levels was very frustrating, and definitely affected my already limited energy levels.

Do you see how when I talk about ableism in occupational therapy I don't just mean in occupational therapy practice? I'd experienced a fair few hurdles before my occupational therapy training had even begun! Why is it that courses, and especially health courses like occupational therapy, have an application process based on systems embedded with such ableism? Being an occupational therapist requires you to have great people skills, not to be an expert mathematician, which felt like the case in my scenario. I fully understand and appreciate that these processes have to be put into place to make things doable, but I bet if an actual occupational therapist was to read these applications to begin with, different decisions would be made. In my personal statement, I spoke about my personal experiences of occupational therapy and how my disability is my tool, and now I've kind of made a career based on this fact!

Experts by experience can improve practice and bring unique skills to the profession. No grade makes a difference to this, and we need to be thinking about this in these early stages. Do we really want a profession full of people who got the same grades at A-Level? People have so much more to bring to the profession to enhance our diversity. We have communities facing serious health inequalities that we need to physically address, so we need people who are prepared to act. And just because you may not have the top grades doesn't mean that you can't go into academia. We have to stop stereotyping and putting people into boxes. As someone who works in academia I am certainly not clued up on everything occupational therapy and I do make mistakes, but that happens, and I can't prevent every mistake I will make. What I *can* do is raise awareness of this to help change the narrative. I have a lot of learning to do, which is why I went into academia because I want to learn more, not because I am all clued up! Of course people who work in academia have a variety of access needs, just like the rest of the population, and we need to make people aware of this. Occupational therapy is such a diverse profession, so let's get on our soapboxes and promote this to the future generation of occupational therapists!

Anyway, back to the story... I had now got my place at university, and although I didn't have the anxieties of leaving home (and neither did my parents), the red tape didn't stop there. A few weeks before receiving my offer from Sheffield Hallam University I began the process of Disabled Students' Allowance (DSA)[2] from Student Finance England.[3] Yet again, this is a long process that has to be done correctly, but my word does it take a lot of energy! Documentation has to be found to 'prove' your disability and needs, and you often have to fill in very lengthy forms, alongside getting a doctor's confirmation of your requirements. My initial assessment for my support plan was around three hours long – three hours! As a disabled person with chronic fatigue this, again, is such an energy drainer in the middle of the lead-up to final A-Level examinations. And not just that – what about mature disabled students who may have jobs and even a family to consider? So much work and planning has to be done to ensure you don't run out of fuel.

The DSA supported me a great deal throughout my degree – well, after we had spent the initial phone call marathon of time to get it set up and sorted, of course. It was still very hard justifying my needs year after year, though, and I often felt judged and got asked if my parents were able to clarify what I was asking from them when I spoke to them via the phone. Why didn't they believe me, but believed my parents, you ask? I think that my speech impairment was the deciding factor here, as it is the most ableist assumption that I face. People make all kinds of assumptions about me when they hear my speech impairment – that I am not competent to make decisions, or even that I am drunk. I am so fortunate that I had my parents throughout the journey as I really wouldn't have got very far without them! In this instance, though, why can't this information be given online?

---

2   www.gov.uk/disabled-students-allowance-dsa
3   https://studentfinance.campaign.gov.uk

These situations increase my internalized ableism, and this is why I have such a big and loud personality. I've always felt the need to tell everyone what I'm doing and what I'm achieving, and this is purely because of the assumptions I have faced. I feel the need to prove myself all the time, and part of me knows I shouldn't feel like this while the other part of me feels the need to show society that disability is not what they perceive it to be. Now I sit here writing this book I'm very glad I chose to be loud as I certainly wouldn't be here today if not. As much as I am proud to be disabled, I do often wonder what my personality would be like if I didn't have cerebral palsy. I know I wouldn't be quiet as I can natter all day, and that certainly is not a disability thing. Would I feel the need to constantly prove myself? I highly doubt it.

I've been told I am inspiring just because I studied to become or have become a disabled occupational therapist. In fact, if I had a pound for every time I heard 'Oh, what an inspiring occupational therapist you'll make', I would be very rich! My experience of disability is that it is a tool and it certainly brings a different dimension to my practice, but it's not inspiring. I went and did my degree following my A-Levels, like many 18-year-olds do. It's simply me just living my life. I get told that I'm inspiring for speaking out and it's greatly humbling to receive these compliments. I don't advocate to make noise, but for the reason behind the noise – it's an integral part of my practice, and I cannot be the occupational therapist I want to be without doing so.

Anyway, point made. Who wants one last ableist story before we round up this chapter?

Oh, it's only the beloved occupational health! Yes, my disabled pals can already feel what's coming.

So my place at university was secure, my DSA was under way, the ball was rolling, and everything was finally happening for me, until occupational health, which was meant to take place in May 2018. However, when I rolled into the appointment with the nurse, it didn't last long before I was told that my situation was 'too complex' and that I needed a doctor. I definitely felt the vibe that they were thinking: 'The disabled girl wants to be an occupational therapist, what? It's unheard of...' Contrary to this nurse's thoughts, I'm really not the first disabled occupational therapist, and nor will I be the last. In actual fact, George Edward Barton, one of the founders of the National Occupational Therapy Society (now known as the American Occupational Therapy

Association), had mental health conditions, an amputation as a result of frostbite and left-hand-side paralysis – all of this while being one of the most influential founding members of various societies and leading theories that we still use in practice in some form today (Christiansen 2017).

So at this nurse's recommendation I went off to see the doctor, and I have never felt so belittled in my entire life. I remember being sat in the room in utter disbelief at the words that were being used, and that it was okay that these words were being said to me (well, it clearly wasn't). I remember being told that I would find this career very challenging, and being given scenarios such as manual handling that I wouldn't be able to do or need support with. In so many words, the doctor told me that I was heading into the wrong profession and would not be able to practice as an occupational therapist. The doctor had an ableist mindset to say the least, and even compared me to other people with cerebral palsy or similar disabilities. This is not okay. Cerebral palsy is an umbrella term (Scope 2022), and no two people with cerebral palsy or any other disability are the same. This is poor practice. I knew it was poor practise back then, but now, having completed my degree, just no! There are no words to describe how wrong this is.

I do understand that the doctor was a medical professional and certainly had more knowledge about placements and practice than I did. But when did it suddenly not become enough to know your own needs as a disabled person? Lived experience is invaluable and needs to be listened to! No one knows how your body works better than you do!

As only an 18-year-old at the time, I believed the doctor, and had a massive anxiety attack. At the time, we, as a family, were already dealing with family trauma, and then the whole process of getting into university was taking its toll, so it's fair to say my mental health was already in quite a state. Receiving this news almost destroyed me and massively provoked my internalized ableism. So much so, that I actually rang up Sheffield Hallam in tears to drop out of the course. The person who picked up the phone was lovely, and along with my mum managed to make me see sense, reassuring me that there was a solution, and that my induction day was the week after, so we should take it from there.

Induction day came and I was a bag of nerves, with the previous week's events still weighing on me. I broke down and cried, all because I couldn't find the room. What a way to impress your future course mates, Georgia!! I was still in the state of mind to quit; everything was too much, and the tears just had to come.

I was saved from making an irrational decision by one of my lovely lecturers, who stopped me in my tracks and asked what was up. I didn't go into detail about occupational health, but just said how things weren't going to plan. My lecturer really helped me in that moment and certainly got me through the morning until I found her and offloaded a few of my worries at lunch (sorry!).

Despite the morning's events I had a great day – I love to natter, so I thoroughly enjoyed meeting new people! At the end of the day I met with that lecturer again and had a conversation about my fears for the course. I say conversation – she actually read my mind about the manual handling worries. Well, I thought she did at the time, but now I know that this is a common situation that many physically disabled healthcare students face. Just like certain placements such as forensic mental health are often ruled out for physically disabled students

She reassured me that my manual handling training wouldn't be an issue and she had already got a plan of what reasonable adjustments needed to go into place under the Equality Act 2010.[4] It was decided that I would do the manual handling on my own first to try it, and then, if I couldn't do it or felt embarrassed, I did not have to attend the training with everyone else. This worked really well. I did attend the training, but it was good to know which ones I didn't feel comfortable with or caused pain so I could take a back step.

I also had a meeting with my fabulous academic adviser and my mum before I started the course, to discuss some of my other concerns (or more so, my worried mother's concerns). These were a list of questions, such as making sure the campus was accessible (yes, that concern didn't just come from mum, and is every wheelchair user's top priority).

My anxiety certainly did take over, but deep down I knew that the doctor at occupational health was wrong; rationally I would have never dropped out even without that lovely lady on the phone that day. Yet the occupational health doctor's words did matter more than they should have, as I was the expert in my needs, and no one else. I knew that doing this degree with my disability was going to be a challenge, but I was up

---

4   www.legislation.gov.uk/ukpga/2010/15/contents

for that challenge as I was pursuing my passion and was ready for the world ahead!

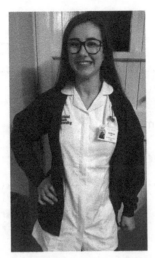

Image 5.2. *Georgia, a white female, stood in her occupational therapy uniform. She is wearing a tunic and a cardigan.*

Ableism within the profession starts from the very beginning and is perpetuated by other systems bigger than the occupational therapy profession itself that need to be challenged. I fully understand that a group of occupational therapists are not going to change the whole university system in the UK, but we have to start somewhere, and as a community full of occupational therapists, surely we are equipped to at least start this conversation to offer disabled students the experience that they deserve?

NOT SO TERRIBLE...P.A.L.S.Y. REFLECTIVE LOG
Pausing
Stop and think about what you have read in this chapter. What are your main takeaway points? What are your main questions?

....

....

....

Analysing

Why did this resonate with you?

....

....

....

Learning

What did you learn from this?

....

....

....

Solving

What actions need to be put into place?

....

....

....

Your plan

How will you achieve these actions? What are your goals?

....

....

....

References

Christiansen, C.H. (2017) 'The architect and his cures – How an eccentric convalescent launched a 100 year old profession.' National Advisory Board Declaration for Independence, 16 March. Accessed on 10 October 2022 at https://declarationforindependence.org/architect-cures-eccentric-convalescent-launched-100-year-old-profession

Scope (2022) 'Cerebral palsy (CP).' Accessed on 27 June 2022 at www.scope.org.uk/advice-and-support/cerebral-palsy-introduction

CHAPTER SIX

Navigating University and Placements with a Disability

This unwelcoming entry to the profession should not carry on, and if a student has a strong desire to go into this area of practice, then reasonable adjustments must be made!

Embarking on your journey at university is nerve-wracking for anyone, never mind when a disability gets thrown into the mix, and there's nothing that I, nor anyone else, can say to fully get rid of those feelings. In this chapter I hope to give you a few tips to help this new world feel a little less scary.

This is going to sound like such a cliché but my biggest worry about going to university was making friends. We all have this worry whether we have a disability or not, but I'd internalized the difficulties from my teenage experiences, and knowing that I was not living in the halls of residence exacerbated these worries. I still wanted a taste of student life; okay, I may not have had the energy to go out as often as others, but I still went out and lived a little. *News flash!* Disabled people like partying and nights out, and they have fun too!

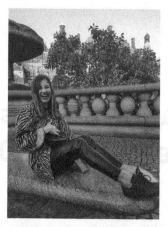

Image 6.1. *Georgia, a white female, wearing a zebra-patterned jacket and leather leggings, sitting on a bench outside. She is goofy-style laughing.*

I know I'm going off topic here, but disabled people know how to have a good time. In the summer of 2018, I went on a girls' holiday and oh my, the amount of people who thought that I was under the influence of illegal substances was shocking. It never occurred to them that a girl with cerebral palsy was out having a good time. Then come the patronizing phrases such as 'good for you' and the utterly disgusting ones such as 'you don't look disabled' or, worst of all, 'you're pretty for a disabled girl' – as well as the comments that my friends got, such as 'well done for taking her out' – I'm sorry, but what even is this supposed to mean?

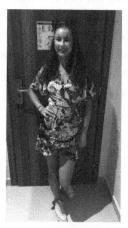

Image 6.1. *Georgia, a white female. The top of her hair is tied up in two space buns and she has glitter on her face. She is wearing a floral dress and has a sparkly bag around her waist.*

I'm sure I don't need to waffle on about how these are not compliments. It would be nice to experience a night out where this doesn't happen or I don't have to show my card to prove I'm disabled with shaky movements and not drunk to get into a nightclub. The 'CP walk' is completely different to the drunk walk, but if you're unsure, then please do educate yourself; society could learn a whole lot from disabled people if they weren't too scared to talk to us!

This brings me on to my first tip for disabled students...

TOP TIP

✓ Network before the course starts, and get to know your future course mates!

Maunder (2017) found that building up social relationships with peers resulted in higher levels of adjustments to university, with these relationships having a crucial impact on transition and belongingness to university. So, after never feeling that sense of belongingness in school that I longed for, I did everything I could to achieve this at university. My first approach to meeting my peers was using social media.

I've said it before and I'm sure I'll say it again, but being active on social media did so many wonders for me, especially in the lead-up to starting university. I accessed a freshers' group for first year students by downloading my university's relevant apps (these will vary according to the course and university), and got to know a few of my course mates. This meant that on the first day of university I felt like I was going to meet friends, as we'd already been talking so much online. I'm not going to pretend that I lived the stereotypical 'fresher's life', because the nights out were kept to a minimum while I was making sure I had enough spoons to fit into my new routine. However, nights out aren't the only way to get to know new friends. I had so many lovely coffee dates with friends during the first semester (well, hot chocolate for me – I'm still not mature enough to drink coffee), and I don't think I missed out on that much while staying at home.

I personally didn't attend that many nights out in my first year (I wish I had done now, seeing as it was illegal to do so in my second and third years, due to the pandemic), and this was for two reasons, the first being that I found I got asked to join a group outing on the day of the event rather than in advance. Not every night out is planned and I've had some great spontaneous nights out, but this is when I've not been busy at university all week! I need to plan so I can save my energy. The second reason was the high level of taxi-related anxiety I had at the time. Taxis are a big part of how I access the world around me, and they were particularly central to my routine before I started using my hand-controlled, adapted car but, at 18 years old, I didn't want to be getting into a taxi solo in the early hours of the morning! Looking back, I think I might have joined in on a few more outings but just returned home earlier than my peers if I was fatigued or in pain. However, I've only gained this new perspective with new-found confidence and experience and through understanding my body's limits more.

You can only do what your body tells you to do.

We certainly push our bodies, and there has been and will be more times when I choose making memories over resting, and that's okay. But we do have to listen to our bodies, and if going out doesn't work for you or isn't even your scene, then don't push yourself to do it. There are plenty of alternative leisure activities such as going to a society or even hanging out virtually if you have limited energy. My campus wasn't far from a park and we had a lovely picnic once to celebrate the end of placement, and they are the memories that I treasure the most!

Knowing your own body's needs is really important to settle into your new environment comfortably. Lots of elements of paperwork are involved in starting university with a disability, such as fire evacuation plans and lots of red tape. Of course this needs to be done, but it's not the most convenient when you just want to get to know your course mates.

Ah, and now here's our old friend disclosure; not only is disclosure a minefield (more to come on this later on), but when you're new to a course and can't predict your future requirements and scenarios, where do you even start? I remember saying, 'it's a case of crossing that bridge when we come to it' so many times during my first few weeks of university, I very much sounded like a broken record! As disabled people, we know that we cannot have knowledge of all our access needs without knowing the environment and role we'll be in, so it's fine to not have all the answers. Yes, we need to be prepared, a lot more prepared than someone who doesn't have as many access needs (remember that everyone has access needs, disabled or not). Sometimes we have to go through the turbulence first to get to the other side, and that is when we'll finally understand the full picture of our requirements in that particular situation.

TOP TIP

✓ Get to know the campus and the accessible routes.

This tip is still not talking about actual studies just yet. Starting university is a huge change for everyone, but particularly a disabled student who may now be in an unknown, less accessible environment, a new city or even country. Are you starting to see how much energy a big change like starting university takes for a disabled person? They may already have chronic fatigue without adding all this to the mix.

Whenever you have a gap in your freshers' week programme, explore all of the new buildings and take your new bestie along. In my opinion, there's no better test of a new friendship than to throw them in the deep end with the palaver of disabled access, a faff that shouldn't still be happening in the 21st century! Jokes aside, though, if you're a young, anxious 18-year-old like I was, then it's best not to do this alone, and I'd certainly ask your academic tutor to support you with this too.

Don't forget to check all the lifts, too, to help you gauge timings on those days when you have a busy schedule. Gauging timings is important as you do not want to be late to a lecture that you are paying for, but it is important to remember that there are always adaptations that can be made and solutions to be found, so don't panic. During my first week of university, I spent about three hours with Disabled Students' Support, waiting to be seen and then going through all of my first semester's timetabled sessions to book assistance to and from my back-to-back classes so I wouldn't be late. It was a painful afternoon (physically and mentally), but I came out feeling a lot more settled about the following weeks at university.

My support lasted a day before I realized it wasn't doing me any favours. I'd miss five minutes of the previous lecture, which costs a whole lot of money and, when I arrived at the next session, the lecturer often wouldn't be there as they'd also had back-to-back teaching. It was ingrained in me to leave classes early as I'd done so ever since I was 12 years old at secondary school. This solution had been found mainly to avoid the school's crowds, but at university there's no avoiding the busy nature of a bustling campus. Plus, I actually felt more comfortable going to and from sessions with people who knew me when having to navigate between lecture buildings. It was much safer to be in a crowd when crossing roads as drivers would be more likely to stop, and you get much more help from friends who know your needs. One road was so inaccessible on my campus that crossing it made me very nervous.

You do have to gauge this and play it by ear – for example, there was an annex behind one building and the wheelchair access was so poor that I needed about ten minutes to get out of the building! Then a further ten minutes to find someone with access to the main building so I could get back on campus. It would have been so much easier if I'd had access to this building on my student ID. These situations are wholly frustrating.

Now we get on to studying, and my biggest tip is...

TOP TIP

✓ Make sure you have a good occupational balance, and learn how to say 'no'!

Going to university offers you so many opportunities in terms of societies, new roles and entertainment in the student union so there really is something for everyone. But sometimes it can be a lot of pressure to get involved with everything. I certainly felt this pressure in my first year, so much so that I ended up seeking counselling to manage my stress and anxiety.

As a disabled person, there's never a boring moment in my life, and just studying for a degree is enough to contend with, but when you add the pressures of navigating everyday life and other general disability-related drama, it easily gets overwhelming. My life had become very busy between assignments and upcoming placements, and I'd also applied to become the disabled students' representative, but, of course, I also had other disability-related drama with getting my adapted vehicle. It was all too much and I ended up being ill as a result of it, so I had to learn to say 'no'. On hearing my counselling psychologist's advice, I decided to give up becoming the disabled students' representative as I was already struggling to find the energy levels to cope.

It was not easy to give it up as I really do love adding my opinions and perspective to roles like this, and I would have gained exciting new experiences such as campaigning. But I made the right decision and was able to focus on my assignments, which leads me to my next tip...

TOP TIP

✓ Don't be afraid to use the support that you're entitled to.

When I started university, I had my learning contract from the university set up as well as my support from DSA[1] through Student Finance England. Both my university and Student Finance England really supported me, but it took me a while to fully utilize my learning contract when applying for things such as extensions on assignments. I really should have used extensions when I needed them right from the start of my degree, as that is what my learning contract was there for. Maybe I didn't use them due to a combination of not wanting to fall behind, my own pride getting in the way or through gaslighting myself – who knows – but I did manage until my final year. Trying to study during a pandemic was tough, and I had no choice but to use the extensions just to keep afloat.

Additionally, the DSA did help a lot during my degree by providing me with my laptop and a specialized, supportive chair alongside other equipment to make studying much easier. Start your DSA application as soon as possible to make sure that you have all your equipment ready when you start your course! Having to navigate processes such as the DSA all my life, I was pretty quick to start all of this as I knew how long it could take. It helped that I had previous experience with disability-related forms. It would have been very easy to miss if I hadn't had this

---

1   www.gov.uk/disabled-students-allowance-dsa

experience and information already, and there are lots of cases where people only get their DSA fully set up a year into studying. Information about how to navigate the DSA should be a lot easier to access but, yet again, it takes a lot of shouting to get something. Be your own advocate and communicate your needs from the beginning to the very end of your university experience!

Another major part of university that needs a whole lot of self-advocacy is the placement system...

Oh look, we've come on to placements – let's open that can of worms and have a nice lovely chat about ableism on placements, as this certainly is an infamous area where ableism strikes.

You'll possibly find that I am missing out on talking about some of the intricacies of university life since I really need to dig my teeth into the whole placement situation. However, there is a fabulous book out there with everything you need to know about this aspect, including how to survive the famous freshers' flu for those party-goers! It also provides more information about living away from home, which I do not have lived experience of.

Check out *University and Chronic Illness: A Survival Guide* by **Pippa Stacey** (2022). It's a really informative read by a phenomenal disabled advocate. I sure wish this book had been published before I embarked on my own university experience.

Finding the right placement is the first hurdle. There are so many areas of this process that are more complicated and messy than necessary due to ableist assumptions. For example, why is it that if you 'can't run', you can't go on a placement in a forensic mental health setting, or if you 'can't kneel', you can't work in paediatrics? The ableism here is just unbelievable! I'll be honest, I wouldn't want to work in forensics anyway as I know my body's limits, but it's unfair that I would be prevented from pursuing this if I chose to. This is such a well-known stigma in the profession and it needs to go. This unwelcoming entry to the profession should not carry on, and if a student has a strong desire to go into this area of practice, then reasonable adjustments must be made!

Reasonable adjustments under Section 20 of the Equality Act 2010[2] are there for a purpose! I know placements don't have the same regulations as being officially employed due to adjustments being made through the DSA and universities, but if you want to be a true ally, then do the homework yourself. Yes, I'll happily use my experience to give advice, but the main essence of this book is to use my experiences to highlight ableism, not to give you a step-by-step guide on how to address and untangle it, because to dismantle any form of discrimination takes collective activism and, most likely, whole new systems need to be created.

I was once given an eight-week placement on a ward. I was admittedly nervous about this and didn't know how my body would cope in this setting. I didn't expect to get denied this kind of placement when I emailed to ask for a pre-placement access review visit. How does an email providing a brief snapshot of my needs give educators everything they need to make a decision to deny me this placement? This is where training is needed to prevent this ableism as, yet again, disabled students are put at a disadvantage through the limited amount of opportunities they have compared to their non-disabled peers. While we are on this topic, universities shouldn't use one singular educator who 'gets it' for all of their disabled students! For example, don't send all of the enquiries to one particular educator who has lived experience of disability rather than to the team as a whole. If occupational therapists can make adjustments and adaptations for the people they serve, then we should be ace at doing this for our colleagues. But we clearly aren't, otherwise I wouldn't have been approached to write this much-needed book.

Navigating placements with a disability is hard, and even my pre-placement visits were something that I hated more and more every time they came around. Despite being hard, pre-placement visits were useful, though, and I was very fortunate that the placement lead where I studied came with me every time, since this provided support and continuity that helped massively. Again, I was asked about my access requirements and what barriers I would face despite being someone who'd never had a job before, let alone had any experience working in practice as an occupational therapist. I knew some of my access needs that would have to be considered, such as not being able to handwrite notes and not being able to stand for very long, but since I'd never been

---

2   www.legislation.gov.uk/ukpga/2010/15/section/20

in any work environment, I didn't know what they needed to know and what adjustments could be provided.

When it came to disclosing my requirements on a pre-placement visit, I always disclosed what *I thought I might need* as I can never be 100 per cent certain of what adjustments I will need as it takes time to get to know the role. Plus, my disability varies from day to day, so I may occasionally need more help on some days.

Placement can be quite frustrating because by the time you figure out what adaptations work for you in that role, the placement is up. You are already fatigued from working daily on placement, and then you end up more fatigued from trying to work out your access requirements. Then your next placement comes in a completely different area of practice, and although you have more of an idea of your needs in practice than before, you're almost back to the drawing board again.

TOP TIP

✓ Always keep a record of the adjustments you've needed in the past.

I had a pre-placement learning agreement with of all the adjustments that I needed on placement, and I just kept updating this during each placement with any additional adjustments I found I needed.

LEARNING AGREEMENT EXAMPLE
Disability: cerebral palsy

I struggle with tasks requiring fine motor skill control, such as writing, cutting up, etc. I am able to write but this may be a slower option, and my writing is hard to understand, so typing is preferred. I may need extra time for notes. I use a laptop for typing and can require additional time for this. I have a voice recorder on my phone if needed.

I struggle to walk for anything further than short distances. I will be able to walk within an area such as an office or seminar room, but would need to use my wheelchair between departments. In the past I have stored my wheelchair in the building

I'm mainly based in when it's not in use, but I do have a hoist in my car now, although I can struggle when independently using this. I drive a heavily adapted vehicle with hand controls.

Previously I have been given my own evacuation plan in the event of a fire. I will require help when setting up equipment that is physically demanding for me. In the past I have told whoever I am with how to do this to demonstrate my understanding without physically setting this up.

I have a speech impairment that is more marked when I am fatigued. My speech can be slurred but is quickly more understandable when the listener is familiar with me. At times I use apps for my speech such as Relay UK for making phone calls and ClaroCom Pro for text-to-speech.

I fatigue easily, although I am confident in managing my own wellbeing and can use breaks if needed to manage my fatigue and pain levels. I can be flexible with my working patterns.

Looking at this now, I'm aware that this is rather negative and focuses on my limitations rather than on how my lived experience of disability enhances my practice. I certainly haven't got everything right, but we can address this and easily change it by developing support plans that are specific to placement and separate to academic work (Health Education England 2022). These need to be put into place and worked on as soon as studies begin, and need to be ever evolving and adaptable. They can then be changed for students, especially those in similar circumstances to what I was in, and for those who have no previous experiences of work and therefore can't predict every access need.

Purple Ella has developed a great tool for disabled students, so do look at her work on Strength-Based Support Plans (Purple Ella 2021).

The *Guide to Practice-Based Learning (PBL) for Neurodivergent Students* by **Health Education England** (2022) also looks at placement-specific support plans, and provides some great tips for both students and practice educators.

Disclosing to a placement educator poses a different dynamic to disclosing to your employer. No matter what the environment is, we must create safe spaces so disabled people can disclose their needs positively to enable them to reach their potential.

During my first few placements I never disclosed my fatigue and used to say to myself 'it's only a few weeks, Georgia, don't moan', when the reality was I wasn't moaning and should have been honest with my educators to get the reasonable adjustments I needed. But disclosing hidden parts of a disability are so much harder, and it was only through the last half of my final placement that I plucked up the courage to be forthcoming about my fatigue. I even faced a big internal battle in doing so on this placement: 'I'm working from home, not even travelling and I still can't do it.' I shouldn't have done this to myself as I was fatigued through juggling my final placement and my dissertation. All of this is a lot for anyone, never mind managing an energy-limiting condition. A safe space must be provided on placement that enables students to disclose positively and not feel judged.

Another fear that links to students not disclosing health conditions is worrying that they won't be believed, as they've possibly previously experienced this from others at some point in their life. This happened to me when on placement. Having been marked down on communication during previous placements and being told that I needed to have some strategies for when people in practice couldn't understand me, I was more than happy to learn about Augmentative and Alternative Communication (AAC). This gave me a great opportunity to enhance my personal and professional development on placement by giving me time to explore which text-to-speech apps were suitable for me. This was greatly appreciated as I was aware that this was something I needed to do after my first placement.

What I wasn't expecting was for my communication to feel like the sole purpose of the placement. I was sat down and told that I needed to see my GP to get referred to speech and language therapy, and that I should speak about this with my parents. I was so taken aback, I went home and told my parents, who said that this was out of line. Deep down, I myself also knew it was wrong, but when you're in that situation and you're being treated like 'just a student', you'll do whatever you need to, to get through. What allowed me to truly realize how ableist this situation had been was when a friend, outside of the disability community, may I add, was speechless when I told her. This then made me reflect on how easy it is to just let ableism slide because of the power imbalance! I got treated as someone who was accessing the occupational therapy services, even though I wasn't because I was too afraid (and had very little energy in the run-up to the winter break) to advocate for myself.

I'm not saying that you shouldn't draw on your unique skillset as an occupational therapist to make adjustments for your students on placement as this skillset should mean you are perfectly placed to do so. However, I was not a service user in this situation, and I had come to placement to learn and enhance my own personal and professional development, not to be referred to speech and language therapy!

The balance shouldn't be so hard to find. But my experience is either that you get treated like a service user or you don't get the reasonable adjustments you need because 'all students should be treated the same'. As occupational therapists, would we treat the people we serve exactly the same, or would we use person-centred practice? I think we all know the answer to that, so why wouldn't we use person-centred practice when working with disabled students and disabled colleagues, as we are all still human beings! A lot of placement-related issues boil down to practice educators thinking that students can be moulded.

Thinking pragmatically, I know that there are restrictions in practice and that practice educators don't get the time they want or need to give students. This can limit their teaching and therefore prevent the student from thriving. But we have to stop putting students into boxes they don't fit in. For instance, going back to the example of AAC, I'm now more motivated to use AAC because I see it as my professional responsibility to meet communication standards set by the Royal College of Occupational Therapists (RCOT) and the Health & Care Professions Council (HCPC), just like you would in any professional role. But is this actually systemic ableism?

For example, take job adverts that read that a candidate 'must show effective verbal and non-verbal communication'; these adverts do not consider those who don't communicate verbally, and the same goes for placement competencies and educators' expectations. Yet again, it comes down to that one line that disabled people are tired of hearing... 'Well, this is the way it's always been done.' That answer doesn't cut it. This is ableist; yes, it might be the way it's always been done, and these competencies might read like this now, but they need to be changed.

How must non-verbal people or those who struggle with written and/or verbal communication feel when they read these competencies or job adverts?

I did eventually use AAC on my final placement so I was supported to use different communication styles and aids. I still got told to work on my 'communication limitations', and that was where the error and ableism was. Yes, I have communication difficulties and I'm not going to deny that, but these are only difficulties because of the barriers I face in society; they are not limitations. Using the phrase 'limitations' suggests that there is a limit that I need to work on and improve, rather than having a speech impairment, which is a fixed difficulty that I experience on a set level that cannot be 'overcome'. You see how much pressure that was?

After dealing with this challenge for two years, still being reminded of this limitation was really getting to me. These everyday microaggressions are what drives my activism the most. I've been disabled all my life and these attitudes don't surprise me and I can take it on the chin, but for someone else who's new to the world of disability, this can really affect them, and it saddens me to think that these experiences may have driven so many amazing occupational therapists out of the profession.

Professional standards must be followed and of course it takes certain characteristics, skills and values to be an occupational therapist, and I'm not saying that every rule needs to be broken. But students shouldn't be made to feel as if they need to be robotic 'mini-educators' to pass the placement. However, as a student I didn't recognize this pressure in terms of my disability, and wouldn't bring any issues related to equity, diversity and belonging (EDB) up. This is a common theme among students. Focus groups with undergraduate occupational therapy students found that if university tutors specifically asked about EDB during the halfway visit, they would be more likely to raise concerns (Graham *et al.* 2022). We therefore need to incorporate this into halfway visits on placement and create a safe space for students.

I do acknowledge that I did have some fabulous experiences on placements, and when my needs were met it worked, but it really does blow my mind that a profession based on the core values and attributes of occupational therapy still can't get this right. Ableism is so prominent in the workplace that it is scary; we all need to be allies and human beings treating students with respect. I know it can be hard being a practice educator while still dealing with the demands of the actual 9–5 job and managing a caseload. Sometimes it's the restraints of practice that are the biggest hurdles, but we know that ableism is systemic and the big hurdles and restraints have to be challenged. For example, on one of my placements they still had handwritten notes, yet I can't legibly handwrite, and so it wouldn't be professional of me to handwrite a person's medical notes – meaning the service I was on placement in had to accommodate my typing of notes instead. They did do this, but my point is that not only is handwriting notes quite uncommon now anyway, it's also obvious that it isn't inclusive. So we need to move with the times and listen to the needs of our incredible workforce, as otherwise we are going to lose them.

It's not easy to challenge this as ableism, and any form of discrimination is learned behaviour – no one is born with these prejudices. But that doesn't mean that students can't challenge it because this is how it starts and we must be given the right tools to do so. I challenged a situation on my final placement, but I only took it further after speaking to my mum about it because I was a student and didn't feel competent enough to do it on my own. I was competent enough, though, and we must empower students to act independently to advocate for themselves by giving them the correct tools. We are all different and we all provide a different perspective, so we shouldn't feel like our experience isn't valued.

There is always a way round things and, as occupational therapists, we can problem-solve and think outside the box; it's in our nature! I'm not expecting perfection, but ableism is unnecessary. If you act as an ally, evaluate your practice and learn from your mistakes just like we all do, we can make placements an enjoyable experience for disabled students.

I've read so many stories about disabled students dropping out of a course because of the ableism they have received both from universities and on placements. Is that the kind of message we want to be giving the people who are the future of our profession? We should be welcoming them with open arms and listening to their stories so that we can act on them, making changes to enhance the diversity and beauty of our wonderful profession.

NOT SO TERRIBLE...P.A.L.S.Y. REFLECTIVE LOG
Pausing
Stop and think about what you have read in this chapter. What are your main takeaway points? What are your main questions?

....

....

....

Analysing
Why did this resonate with you?

....

....

....

Learning
What did you learn from this?

....

....

....

Solving
What actions need to be put into place?

....

....

....

Your plan
How will you achieve these actions? What are your goals?

....

....

....

References

Graham, M., Bacha, S., Martinez, E. and Vine, G. (2022) 'Feeling Connected: Exploring Equity, Diversity and Belonging with Undergraduate Occupational Therapy Students.' Paper Presentation. Royal College of Occupational Therapists 45th Annual Virtual Conference, June.

Health Education England (2022) *Guide to Practice-Based Learning (PBL) for Neurodivergent Students*. Accessed on 12 February 2023 at www.hee.nhs.uk/ sites/default/files/documents/Guide%20to%20Practice-Based%20Learning%20 %28PBL%29%20for%20Neurodivergent%20Students.pdf

Maunder, R.E. (2017) 'Students' peer relationships and their contribution to university adjustment: The need to belong in the university community.' *Journal of Further and Higher Education 42*, 6, 756–768. Accessed on 20 December 2022 at https:// doi.org/10.1080/0309877X.2017.1311996

Purple Ella (2021) 'Strength Based Support Plans – Disability.' [Video] 14 May. Accessed on 22 December 2022 at www.youtube.com/watch?v=ctJ6KDVy4P8

Stacey, P. (2022) *University and Chronic Illness: A Survival Guide*. Barton-upon-Humber: Daisa & Co. Accessed on 3 August 2022 at www.lifeofpippa.co.uk/product/university-and-chronic-illness-a-survival-guide-by-pippa-stacey

CHAPTER SEVEN

My Virtual Role-Emerging Placement

I was so incredibly lucky that Margaret came to visit me that day, as she has had such a massive impact on my professional career.

Now I know what you're thinking, we know you did a virtual placement, Georgia – most occupational therapists who studied throughout the pandemic did the same! We've all read the stories, I know. Yet my virtual placement would have taken place in 2020, pandemic or no pandemic. This chapter will be discussing the ableism in why it took a global pandemic to highlight a need that the disabled community have been fighting towards improving for a very long time. So let's get into the story, shall we?

One of the reasons I was drawn to study at Sheffield Hallam University is that it included a role-emerging placement, and not every university that I had applied for had this option. For those less familiar with occupational therapy, a role-emerging placement happens when a student has a placement in a non-traditional area of practice that doesn't currently have an occupational therapist in post. All the posts in the NHS and social services began as role-emerging. To illustrate how this process works, the student/s have to work within and assess the placement, scoping it to identify an occupational area of need for the people within the service, and work together to create a therapeutic intervention, programme or package. It is also referred to as an 'extended scope placement', as you 'scope out' or review areas of clinical need and develop an intervention to be delivered within your placement.

I was really intrigued to find out more about this type of placement and was looking forward to this area of my studies the most, as I felt I could utilize my transferable skills. Although the placement was halfway through my studies, it was certainly on my mind a lot as far back as the beginning of the course. Disabled people often have to plan any activity or workplace scenario well in advance, to be able to structure this around our needs and access requirements. My traditional placements also needed additional planning but were more straightforward to plan as I was getting used to the traditional student–educator dynamic, so it was easier to establish my needs in these situations. Knowing I wouldn't have a practice educator by my side on my role-emerging placement certainly did increase my anxiety, although things became less uncertain and anxious for me when my link tutor, Margaret Spencer, came to visit me halfway through my first placement.

Margaret Spencer is the largest provider of occupational therapy supervision in the UK, and has over 30 years' experience providing supervision, from newly qualified occupational therapists to commissioners and case managers. Margaret is the most creative person I have ever met and is definitely an occupational therapist through and through. I was so incredibly lucky that she came to visit me that day, as she has had such a massive impact on my professional career. We still work very closely today, including the 'making' of this book. Let's just say that when Margaret and I get together, we intend to make waves, and the bigger the wave, the better.

At the time I had only come across Margaret once before at university, so we didn't know each other. So on the visit, as well as asking me all the standard questions that the visit entailed, she took the time to get to know me and find out my personal attributes. It's great to remind ourselves that our personal and social attributes make us the therapists that we are!

One of the questions she asked me was about what area of occupational therapy practice I would like to go into when I finalized my studies. I replied that paediatrics was my current focal area, but I also said how open I was to exploring different areas of practice, as occupational therapy is so broad. The conversation flowed on (surprising what you can fit into 45 minutes), and I mentioned how I loved blogging and had my own blog named *Not So Terrible Palsy*[1] that I would love to write more occupational therapy content on, and, as Margaret put it, 'the seed was then sown'.

---

1   https://notsoterriblepalsy.com

I had only started my blog three months prior to this conversation so it was in its infancy and lacked a full-scale amount of professional content. Due to this, it was not something I often brought up in conversations. However, my supervisor asked me to do my end of placement presentation about my blog (okay, so maybe I did bring it up sometimes, but it was a community placement, and a lot of time was spent with my educator in the car). This wasn't the case study presentation that I was expecting and it sparked my motivation to mention my passion for blogging to Margaret...best decision I ever made!

During that visit, we started discussing plans for my role-emerging placement that would start ten months later. I felt such a huge relief not having to initiate plans about it. Margaret gave me a challenge instantly: to incorporate more occupational therapy content into *Not So Terrible Palsy*. So I did, and a few weeks later the first post and my first occupational therapy blog was launched – 'Why I study occupational therapy' – even though the placement was nine-and-a-half months away.

We met back in university in September and sketched out a few rough plans (I still have the image of the notes we wrote on a scrap piece of paper). With the beginning of my second year now starting, plans were well and truly underway, and I used my planning time as part of the scoping exercise and was able to record a few placement hours that September before the placement started. The flexibility that Margaret enabled me to have here regarding my hours meant so much to me! The World Federation of Occupational Therapists (WFOT) sets the standard that students must complete 1000 hours of clinical placements to qualify as an occupational therapist, but did you know that there is little research to support this actually being a beneficial set amount of developmental placement time?

Where is the equity? How inequitable that chronically ill students are expected to do the same amount of hours as others without a disability. We all know how tiring placement is: learning a new role, the constant pressure of being observed, the new routine, keeping up with studies and writing up weekly reflections. It's hard work for any student, never mind those who have to deal with fatigue or other energy-sapping symptoms such as pain or sickness just from going about their normal day-to-day. The flexibility Margaret allowed me when filling out my placement hours made such a difference to my functional body.

I do understand why clinical placement is important, believe you me, and, in terms of my own personal and professional confidence, I would have loved to have been out on placement a lot more prior to heading into my first role. But no matter how many clinical hours you have on placement, you're never going to feel competent when you walk into your first post.

Having Margaret, who got to know and understand me and how I worked so well, as my supervisor for this placement was a big weight off my shoulders. I fully appreciate time is rarely given for reflective practice in the 9–5 job, yet having this time on placement did wonders in helping me to identify myself as a thriving occupational therapist. The role of an occupational therapist is so much more diverse and flexible than what happens during the 9–5 job. Our perception of the role becomes this as we are only presented with the delivery of our placement in 9–5 placement hours, and I speak here not to challenge but as an advocate for our profession. Of course, these placements are unable to showcase the huge array of roles a real-world occupational therapist can pursue, yet showcasing this very narrow, limited viewpoint of occupational therapy and tasks that were incredibly physically and fatigue-inducing definitely triggered my internalized ableism. There are so many parts of being an occupational therapist that I struggle less with, such as reflective practice (in case my 60,000-word book didn't give you that impression). Everyone's skillset is different – mine just also happens to include my modified abilities – but placements on a reduced timescale give disabled students no opportunity to modify their experience and thrive as they would in the real world of practice. My role as an occupational therapist is not solely defined by the structures of my 'clinical' practice; it is me using occupational therapy theory in everything I do, like using my knowledge right now as I type... The occupations of an occupational therapist – that's one to fry our brains, isn't it?

I hope I have been able to explain why this chapter was so crucial to the book. This isn't just another virtual placement story – we planned this and started it well before we even knew about the pandemic, and it was one of the first, if not the first, in the UK. Part of the placement included numerous virtual calls nationally and internationally to explain how we had created the virtual placement. Having had this unique opportunity and realizing what it brought to my ability to demonstrate all the competencies required of the professional body without the confines of the 9–5 placement, I wanted to use it to show how creative and innovative we can be as therapists, if we allow ourselves to think outside of the conventional box that many disabled people cannot function properly inside of. I've said it before and I'll certainly say it again...this is about fighting for something that the disabled community have been fighting for, for decades. Give us some flexibility and let us demonstrate how we can provide a new prism through which to view the world.

This leads me on to why the information-gathering stage of the occupational process was so crucial for the placement, as illustrated by Creek (2014).

Information gathering

After many discussions, we finally had an idea of what my virtual placement was going to look like. The main idea was that I was going to use my blog to raise awareness of online communities and the power of online tools for those who found it difficult to leave the house – let's get on my soapbox again!

The idea for the placement was inspired by my friend Francesca, who I met online. Fran brought the power of online networks for disabled people to my attention back in 2018, and although I was immediately interested to explore the topic, I kept quiet as I knew that Fran had taken this concept to the BBC Young Reporters Competition (BBC News 2019). I knew this because I played a small part in it, aiding Fran in filming her report and meeting her in person for the first time. What an experience that was, not only to meet Fran but also to get the opportunity to help her highlight such an important topic!

Fran went on to win the competition, which only made my interest in this subject matter stronger. I'd only been at university a few months when Fran and I met. I still had a long way to go before finishing my degree, but I now had more than a basic understanding of occupational therapy. I understood that engaging in online communities and social media was an occupation in itself, and Fran's report highlighted that this was an occupation that made her feel less 'isolated' and 'alone' as a disabled person, removing barriers. Occupational deprivation is defined as a 'a state of preclusion from engagement in occupations of necessity and/or meaning due to factors that stand outside immediate control of the individual' (Whiteford 2000, p.201). Chronic fatigue and pain is out of our control and, yes, there are times when I've not been able to go out as often as I'd wanted to; I try to plan around my health, but some days that doesn't work. Although I was not as knowledgeable on concepts such as 'occupational deprivation' when I first met Fran, I could see the powerful influence that online platforms had within the disabled community. These not only advocate for disability rights, but also address isolation, despite the impact of 'occupational isolation' not being well known within the occupational therapy community. I only felt confident to identify as a disabled person and less alienated because of the online communities, so I knew that I had to be the one to raise awareness of the importance of these in the world of occupational therapy.

The idea to raise awareness of online networks for the disabled community just kept getting bigger, as we also wanted to explore online networks as a whole within the profession, and alternative online options for people like myself. As I've mentioned, my disability meant that juggling placements, assignments and fatigue levels had always been particularly challenging, yet working from home allowed me to manage everything a lot better and have a greater occupational balance. This is another way that traditional placements are failing the disabled student community, as remote working certainly meets my needs far better in every way.

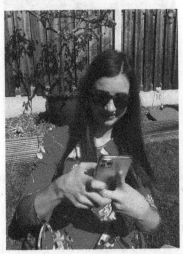

Image 7.1. *Georgia, a white female, sat in a garden on her phone. She is wearing sunglasses and a floral dress.*

The facts

Meaningful occupation increases our wellbeing (Duncan 2021), although another essential factor to this is our environment. The environment plays an enormous role in determining our occupational performance. I know that working from home allowed me to get the most out of my placement.

Working in my home environment allowed me to be more comfortable on placement. For example, I was able to have my own specialized chair, which resulted in me experiencing less pain from my cerebral palsy while working. I was therefore able to be more productive, getting more work done without pain distracting me, and this enhanced my overall occupational performance on placement, as I could work productively and independently, thus improving my wellbeing (Duncan 2021).

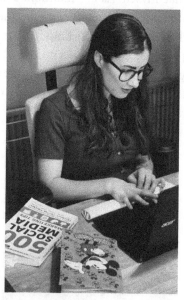

Image 7.2. *Georgia, a white female, sat in a custom computer-style chair. She is working on her laptop and has books around her.*

Do you see how important working from home is? I know I can be a lot more productive when I don't have to get up at the crack of dawn and rush around getting washed, dressed, my hair and make-up done to get to work – this increases my fatigue and pain levels, especially when I am travelling somewhere. I understand that not everyone likes remote working and that face-to-face contact cannot be replaced, but why was this alternative not being offered to disabled students before the pandemic? We established earlier on in this book that not every clinical skill can solely be learned through a clinical environment!

My placement also highlighted the need for virtual healthcare, which was a huge point I've been wanting to address for a very long time! I can't tell you how many times I've attended a medical appointment at the other end of the city, lost many hours of my education, to be told 'we'll see you next year' after 15 minutes. Again, I am a chronically ill person with a very small pot of energy, and surely this energy could be used more wisely? This affects the whole family dynamic when you're rushing around to get to an appointment at 9 am; of course, medical appointments have priority, but we still have other occupations and responsibilities to carry out!

My placement had only had the national and international reach it did because of the COVID-19 pandemic. The question had to be asked, why did it take a global pandemic for the world to finally realize these benefits for disabled people, after years of the disabled community advocating for this?

After completing the placement, I went on to get published in the *Young Voices* section of *BMJ, Paediatrics Open*, where I discussed my experiences in a piece titled 'Benefits of online healthcare if one has a disability' (Vine 2020).

I think I had enough information to get on with my assessment – do you?

Assessment

The assessment part of the occupational therapy process involved weekly blogging – initially asking the disabled community what exactly the online community meant to them. At the time, it was a few weeks before we went into lockdown, and I did get some mixed reactions towards the placement and its purpose, and I was aware of this. Which is why preparing for the first blog post to go live was *so* nerve-wracking – I had never been so scared for a blog post to go live before. What if people didn't understand what I was trying to communicate? What if this was not the right time to launch the project? I had so many questions but they would not answer themselves until the blog post went live. I am certainly a lot more ruthless now!

The reaction to the blog was incredible and overwhelming. Although the reaction was truly humbling, it made me evaluate *Not So Terrible Palsy* and its purpose. Prior to this placement I was just posting blogs for the sake of it, but from then on, I realized my motivations and my staunch passions towards tackling ableism within healthcare. This driving force to tackle ableism only grew as the placement progressed!

Intervention

A few weeks into my placement I received an email from Occupational Therapists Without Borders (OTWB),[2] who had noticed my blogs and were interested in my virtual placement. They asked if I was interested in volunteering with them. OTWB is a group of occupational therapists, students, occupational therapy assistants and other healthcare professionals who promote the profession in low- and middle-income countries, and it was the platform I needed to make sure my voice was being heard.

Knowing the global impact that OTWB has on the profession, I was more than up for volunteering with them and getting my content there. I was expecting them to want a blog or two about my virtual placement, and that was all. What I was not expecting was for them to email me back a few days later offering me the title 'digital production director and global students ambassador'. Me? A girl from Sheffield, with such a title – I could not believe it. But as part of my placement, I seized the opportunity (that's what people on placements do), and working with OTWB has been incredible. I have learned so much from connecting with occupational therapists around the world. OTWB is now an Affiliate Member of the Occupational Therapy Africa Regional Group and the World Federation of Occupational Therapists (WFOT), so I am very excited about what future work with OTWB may look like. I do know that there is going to be a whole lot more disrupting from my perspective moving forward.

Eventually we had done it; all those hours Margaret and I had spent

---

2   https://designdn.wixsite.com/otwb/about

planning were worth it, as we had exceeded our initial aims and gained not only a national but also an international reach. We were collaborating with OTWB and had also been noticed by occupational therapists from Australia and Canada, who connected with us on a Saturday morning online, such is the power of the virtual community. We also hosted a *#OTalk* on disclosure (Spencer and Vine 2020), and found that disclosure and auditing humanizing experiences in a clinical setting can enhance the therapeutic relationship when done correctly, as occupational therapists are not robots, and both parties benefit from the relatable experience.

This was only a month into the three-month placement, and there are so many more stories I could write in this chapter. But what's the point if we don't look at what this actually meant for the disabled community? Did this tackle ableism and address the importance of online platforms for the disabled community?

Evaluation

Okay, we do have one more story from the placement to tell before I can round this chapter off. The evaluation of my placement came from the webinar. Do you see how I did an end of placement presentation that demonstrated my use of the occupational therapy process just like any other placement? It's really not that hard to make an accessible placement!

The webinar took a lot of planning and I was very stressed during that time, as back then webinars were a big deal rather than being a regular part of your CPD (continuing professional development). Not to mention I obviously had the communication competency on my mind again, since I have a speech impairment due to my cerebral palsy! Given my last placement in assistive technology, I did use and accept AAC this time. I had fully manually recorded from my laptop as I was still convinced I didn't need the AAC app I use currently, but at the time it was a big step towards modifying my experience to suit my needs.

The webinar was streamed on YouTube, so occupational therapists around the globe could join to hear about the importance of online communities, and although it wasn't highlighted then, we discussed the clearly ableist perspective and learning channels in the profession. I wish I'd taken a different approach in the presentation and the whole placement so I could be more clear about the fact that I wanted to challenge the ableist view of not recognizing online communities as a meaningful occupation. This always happens to every student on a role-emerging placement. Once the placement is completed, they know exactly where they would start if they were doing that placement again – that's the learning! Qualifying as an occupational therapist was important to me, but this limited the amount of challenging that took place on my part, and it's taken me a while to realize this fact. Now I am qualified and am free to get on with the job I started with the knowledge, skills and abilities I gained from my role-emerging placement.

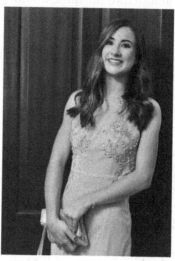

Image 7.3. *Georgia, a white female, in a ball dress with her hair and make-up done (this was Georgia's profile at the time, and the face of advertising for the webinar).*

This version of the chapter you are reading is completely different to my first draft, where I literally talked you through the whole placement. This chapter is actually about what this placement taught me; it has shaped me with the content of my blogs and helped to define the occupational therapist I am today. This unique placement opportunity allowed my blog to find its niche and for me to find my passion of challenging ableism. Of course, I talked about disability prior to this placement on my blog, but there is a whole world of brilliant disabled advocates out there, and I was a very small fish in a very big pond. I still float around occasionally and do not quite know where I am going, although I've grown as a person and blogger, so my pond seems a lot smaller now.

Formulating this placement took a lot of work and we did more foundation laying than disrupting; however, I still wouldn't change anything we did. The end of my virtual placement was the start of my career in this profession, and we made a huge step in getting occupational therapists to read words written by the disabled community.

We still have a long way to go, but this placement gave me the platform that I needed. The goal was for me to link my disabled activism skills with my occupational therapy skills, and that's what we achieved, with bells on! I use my disabled activist skills every single day at work when I'm the occupational therapist, as it would be impossible for me to be in this profession without doing so.

So, in terms of reducing ableism, my virtual role-emerging placement didn't change much, and even the #OTalk on disclosure would have some very different questions now. However, like all role-emerging placements it's a start, and it has got me to where I am, writing this book to challenge ableism, and for that I will forever be thankful for the placement we created. Now I definitely know my purpose as an occupational therapist, and my role and responsibility as a disruptor and disabled advocate.

NOT SO TERRIBLE...P.A.L.S.Y. REFLECTIVE LOG

Pausing
Stop and think about what you have read in this chapter. What are your main takeaway points? What are your main questions?

....

....

....

Analysing
Why did this resonate with you?

....

....

....

Learning

What did you learn from this?

. . . .

. . . .

. . . .

Solving

What actions need to be put into place?

. . . .

. . . .

. . . .

Your plan

How will you achieve these actions? What are your goals?

. . . .

. . . .

. . . .

References

BBC News (2019) 'BBC young reporters share their stories.' [Video] 6 March. Accessed on 16 October 2022 at www.bbc.co.uk/news/41366824

Creek, J. (2014) 'Approaches to Practice.' In J. Creek, W. Bryant, J. Fieldhouse and K. Bannigan (eds) *Creek's Occupational Therapy and Mental Health* (6th edn) (pp.50–71). Glasgow: Elsevier.

Duncan, E.A.S. (2021) *Foundations for Practice in Occupational Therapy* (6th edn). Edinburgh: Elsevier.

Spencer, M. and Vine, G. (2020) 'Experiences of the journey from service user to a professional.' *#OTalk*, 24 March. Accessed on 16 October 2022 at https://otalk. co.uk/2020/03/17/otalk-april-21st-april-experiences-of-the-journey-from-a-service-user-to-a-professional

Vine, G. (2020) 'Benefits of online healthcare if one has a disability.' *BMJ Paediatrics Open, Young Voices 4*, 1, 1–2. Accessed on 2 January 2023 at https://bmjpaedsopen. bmj.com/content/4/1/e000851

Whiteford, G. (2000) 'Occupational deprivation: Global challenge in the new millennium.' *British Journal of Occupational Therapy 63*, 5, 200–204. Accessed on 21 April 2023 at https://doi.org/10.1177/030802260006300503

CHAPTER EIGHT

Calling Out Ableism in Occupational Therapy Studies

We need to stop sugar-coating the profession; overall I've had some amazing experiences, but the profession has its flaws.

So I made it to the final year of university. I was almost there, my completed degree was within touching distance. Going into my final year, I felt so empowered having just done my virtual placement. I was ready for my dissertation proposal, my final placement and to start job hunting! It was sad knowing that my final year would be through virtual study due to the pandemic, especially considering how close my cohort were. Due to the in-person nature of an occupational therapy course, I originally thought that we would have hands-on training in a simulated healthcare setting. Yet in the end, our mandatory training certificate got extended and everything transitioned to being online. This was a bittersweet feeling as my anxiety surrounding in-person attendance disappeared, and knowing that my course mates and I would never all be in a lecture theatre again was sad. But we made the best of the situation and had a few virtual coffees to lift spirits.

Despite the strange circumstances, working from home suited my access needs, so I soon got into the new routine. It frustrates me that some work environments have already reverted to solely face-to-face working since the pandemic, when working remotely meets the access needs of many disabled people, including students. To get the best out of us, listen to our access needs. We don't invent our access needs just because we want to work in our pyjama bottoms!

> **Sam Pywell** (2021) researched the request to dial in to make lectures and seminars more accessible through online study for disabled students. Sam often references this need for inclusion during her conference presentations.

However, working online did pose its challenges; 'Zoom fatigue' is real and certainly was for me as someone who fatigues easily. I also quickly became quite self-conscious when speaking on virtual video platforms, especially when I was among unfamiliar people. From being marked down on my communication on previous placements, I was becoming more self-conscious than I'd ever been about my speech impairment. Therefore, if I was online speaking to a group of new people, I would choose to type my responses and often, by the time I'd typed in the chat, the moment had been and gone!

My communication is still quite a sensitive subject for me. Yes, I'm a lot more open to using AAC now through written communication or using the text-to-speech function. If I am giving a presentation with advanced notice, I will, nine times out of ten, use AAC as I know when I'm presenting that this will save me energy. AAC is a fantastic aid, especially when I am fatigued, yet it does take more time to prepare, and the process itself can be tiring.

I recognize my privilege to have the option of both verbal and non-verbal communication. We're all allowed to feel confused at times, though, and I'm still figuring out my journey with AAC. As I write this, I'm currently preparing for my postgraduate certificate (PGCert) to become a qualified lecturer in occupational therapy. Therefore, I still have barriers to face around how I will manage this in the future, and I know it will take a bit of reflecting.

Throughout this journey, I will need allies to be patient with me and to accept that I might decide to use the chat feature in virtual meetings instead of speaking. In my final year of university, a lecturer who didn't know me decided to call me out in an online lecture for not verbally speaking! Yes, this is wrong, but the situation was resolved and we had a meeting. To me it was just another reminder of the daily barriers and misconceptions surrounding disabled people. This is why disabled students face so many hurdles at university.

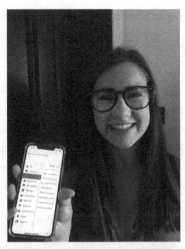

Image 8.1. *Georgia, a white female, with dark hair and glasses, shown here holding her phone, which showcases her text-to-speech app. This has many different categories and phrases, but the text at the top reads 'Hello, my name is Georgia'.*

During my final year, I found everything so hard – of course the pressure and expectation increases in the final year, but for me it wasn't the pressure itself; it was balancing all this, and it weighed on me quite heavily in terms of my mental health. I'd been balancing this for two years – why, all of a sudden, couldn't I do it? This showed in my assignment grades too. Of course the assignments got harder, but I'd started off the academic year being able to make this jump, yet by semester two I was struggling to keep afloat. So much so that when I was in a tutorial and my academic tutor asked how I was, I just burst into tears, and it's still one of those moments that I don't know where it came from. There was no building up to it; in fact, I actually remember feeling more frustrated in that session because we'd presented a group project that didn't go to plan. But no, as soon as I answered my academic tutor's question, the flood gates opened. This then increased my internalized ableism – if I couldn't manage this, then how was I going to manage the working world? I'm not saying it's not okay to cry – crying is good and it's clearly what I needed in that moment. I was just so confused and deflated that I couldn't manage what I'd managed before. It's not as though I didn't have the time – we had to stay at home after all!

Luckily, after a few more wobbles and not bad but unusually low grades for myself, my final placement came to an end in the spring and everything became a bit easier. I still had a few wobbles, for example

I could request to repeat an assignment if I felt like I was not in the best place to get the highest grade I could attain. Therefore, with my mental health not being the best due to stress, pain and fatigue levels, I requested to repeat two of my upcoming assignments. This was denied, which is fine – it's not all about grades and yes, a lot of this pressure was coming from myself. However, it was frustrating when this was denied, especially when I was already at a low point and I did consider repeating the year. Maybe I would have been better at balancing this the second time around? What did reassure me was the amount of support I received from my personal tutor and the academic team.

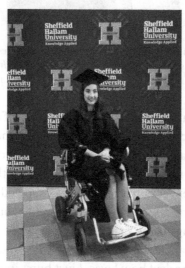

Image 8.2. *Georgia, a white female, sat in her cap and gown at graduation in her electric wheelchair. There's a board behind her advertising the university, which repeats the phrase 'Sheffield Hallam University Knowledge Applied'.*

A lot of the people I meet now, whether this be through work or my own experiences of being a service user, say 'I bet you got a first class degree.' Yes, I did, and I am privileged academically and I understand that there are others out there who work their butt off and still don't attain their desired grade, whatever that may be. But I don't think people realize how much energy it took me as a chronically ill person through a pandemic to achieve that. Yes, I pushed myself and I probably could have achieved a 2:1 more comfortably because my grades two months prior to finishing did not indicate a first class degree, I'll tell you that. I'm not saying it's easy for anyone because it's not, but my passion motivated me to push myself because my chronically ill body was certainly ready to give up on studying.

Even though as a disabled student I had more to contend with, I was not alone, which massively motivated me, and I do have to say that the academic team did their best to keep our spirits up during lockdown. This compassion from our tutors was so important and is needed, pandemic or no pandemic.

Although I struggled in my final year as someone who crumbled under the pressure of exams, I was ecstatic to find out that passing my degree wouldn't be determined in this way but instead through written assignments. Others with different learning needs may find assignments hard – there are other ways to evidence learning aside from assignments and presentations, and we need to play to students' strengths.

Dr Mandy Graham, a reader in occupational therapy, explores inclusion within academia from the perspective of both a lecturer and someone who herself has access needs in her piece 'Thriving, not surviving, with dyslexia':

> Like many people with invisible disabilities, I wasn't diagnosed with dyslexia until later in life (Murphy and Stevenson 2018); aged 39 and halfway through my PhD! As a Senior Lecturer in Occupational Therapy at the time, some might find my career path surprising, given the challenges with writing, spelling, multi-tasking and information processing that is commonly associated with the specified learning difficulty (Falzon 2021). However, it was being in an academic role that brought things to light, opening doors to the full assessment process, a reasonable adjustment plan, funding from a Disabled Student Allowance (DSA), access to a learning support tutor, and relevant software. I was now as such, on the other side of the fence, realizing my unique contribution.
>
> My preferred learning style has always been visual and kinaesthetic; utilizing creative approaches such as diagrams, images, infographics, video, music, animation, role plays, use of colour coding, 3D models and interactive engagement. Such multi-sensory strategies I now understand are typically helpful for adults with dyslexia (Dobson Waters and Torgerson 2021), in addition to technology (Pino and Mortari 2014) which I often use within my teaching to stimulate debate, encourage sharing of ideas, and to recap knowledge via polls, platforms and quizzes.
>
> Conversely, offering choice within assessment is a hotly debated

topic, with flexibility and inclusivity essential to widening participation in higher education (Falzon 2021). Yet I often reflect, would I be where I am without having learnt to adapt and develop my own tactics to pedagogical approaches of the 1990s? Would I have been able to write concise, formal reports for Mental Health Review Tribunals, recall and apply complex information on the spot in fast paced acute environments, and have developed the resilience and determination required in an ever-changing NHS, if I had always chosen the method of assessment aligned to my strengths? This notion of intended personal growth is supported by the need for Continued Professional Development (CPD) throughout our careers as occupational therapists in order to meet the complexities of emerging practice (WFOT 2016) and evolve as effective allies (Atwal, Sriram and McKay 2021). Hence, a universally designed yet varied curriculum should be balanced with support to celebrate diversity and realize potential to enable all students to thrive within higher education.

I know that different universities have different support systems in place, and I'm not denying that the current support isn't useful. Focus groups made up of undergraduate students showed that they liked being challenged, with students reporting that challenging assignments allowed them to leave their comfort zone and gain skills that are useful in practice (Graham *et al.* 2022). I'm not recommending that students choose their assignments every time as this gives variety and challenge to them, preparing for practice. Also, this poses more challenges such as issues for markers and ensuring that assignments meet professional requirements. But it's about being flexible and open to different processes when structural changes do happen. We continually need to ask ourselves, is there any way we can make assessments more accessible in order to meet a variety of different learning needs?

The pitfall here is that universities struggle to individualize their courses due to cultural and institutional barriers, preventing students from achieving a sense of belonging (Thomas 2022). Again, this is because discrimination is systemic and the practicalities just aren't there for flexibility within occupational therapy courses. The power to change this comes from a higher level and therefore needs to be considered by both universities and the overarching occupational therapy community.

Dr Dave S.P. Thomas's 'Belonging matters', written for Black History Month 2022, is a must-read to enhance our understanding of belongingness and allyship, particularly for students (Thomas 2022).

As Dr Thomas (2022) writes, 'the benefits of a diverse workforce (including those with visible or non-visible markers of diversity) and a diverse society are widely accepted', and I couldn't agree more. Not only does this enhance the diversity of the profession in terms of thinking about clinical practice, it also aligns with the *NHS Long Term Plan* (NHS 2019) in ensuring that we represent those we serve. Given that I have little experience of clinical practice, I would be a bag of nerves walking into a clinical role. But I know that in the past, when I've used my 'diverse markers' (Thomas 2022) on placement and therapeutic use of self, it has benefited my relationship with the individual I'm working with.

Belongingness is an intrinsic motivation to be socially accepted within our community or group (Pillow, Malone and Hale 2015). Different individuals find community in different ways; personally, I found an active online community that I belong with and that helped me form my identity as a disabled activist. Belonging-centred practice helps to identify the needs within a social group or occupation (Whalley Hammell 2014), just like I have done through the disabled community. Joining this community has enabled me to not only be confident in my own body, but has also given me such a sense of belonging that it is my drive behind every single piece of work that I do. Occupational therapists have the tools to look at occupational participation among communities and address the social and economic determinants (Malfitano, Whiteford and Molineux 2019). *When practice instead focuses on community, interdependence and belonging, society is then represented in a realistic manner.*

A research assignment at university allowed me to focus on a local community and reflect on how this mirrored the marginalized individuals within this social group. Focusing on a group rather than an individual allowed me to analyse these systemic injustices across society as a whole. An overall trend currently is that practice is becoming more belonging-centred. Hortop (2022) suggests that belonging-centred practice shifts the focus from the individuals to their belonging groups, reinstating interdependence. Furthermore, Iwama (2006) explains that 'there is greater value in "belonging" and 'interdependence" than in unilateral agency' (Whalley Hammell 2014, citing Iwama 2006, p.155).

In higher education, belongingness is essential to provide a feeling of connection to the institution and campus community (Pedler, Willis and Nieuwoudt 2021). This belongingness therefore increases academic attainment as students then have more positive feelings towards the university and will be more likely to get involved (Pedler *et al.* 2021). And to enhance belongingness you need a compassionate environment.

Lack of compassion can have significant effects on student engagement, often resulting in unproductive teamwork, silences, stress and certain students monopolizing the class (Brentnall and Stanbury 2023). I, personally, was quite confident to have a go at answering questions in class, but there were still times that I found engagement hard. For example, on placements, I would go for weeks without speaking to course mates, due to lack of energy to socialize while managing the placement. That meant that sometimes when returning to campus it would take us a while to break that ice and work as a team again within seminars. Using my experiences of working in academia, I can now see that there are all sorts of reasons why this engagement decreases, which are not just disability or placement related. There can be an array of reasons why students lack belongingness to their course. Therefore, compassionate pedagogies such as Cooperative Learning Interaction Patterns (CLIPS)[1] can be used in an interactive way to enhance group work and engagement, resulting in students feeling empowered (Werdelin Education 2019), and like they belong.

Motivation, enjoyment and, of course, personal factors also impact belongingness (Pedler *et al.* 2021). To me, an important factor that increased my sense of belongingness was having student membership to the Royal College of Occupational Therapists (RCOT) as that gave me an identity. As a student, I was lucky enough to have the funds for my RCOT membership provided by my university, which greatly influenced my decision to join and engage more with the professional body. The cost of membership is a barrier to most students, even more so for those with energy-limiting conditions who can't work while studying. Having

---

1   CLIPS are a series of content-free action steps that micro-manage how learners interact with each other and teaching materials.

to fund this without even knowing how worthwhile membership would be to them individually weighs heavily on this decision. Research with undergraduate students shows that if higher education institutions provided the funds for RCOT membership, students would be more likely to join (Graham *et al.* 2022).

Financial pressures while managing a degree are hard, and this is why it is important to have separate spaces that don't charge for membership, such as AbleOTUK.[2] I am proud to be a founding member of this affinity group. When I was a student, AbleOTUK wasn't established and I would spend a lot of time finding occupational therapy students like myself to connect with. Now having AbleOTUK as a known affinity group enhances engagement further by providing online monthly safe spaces for people within the profession who have lived experience of disability to connect.

Connecting with occupational therapists from different backgrounds was important to me because, due to barriers in education, there aren't enough diverse professionals out there. Some professionals with protected characteristics may also choose to be less visible due to their previous negative experiences being internalized. This then perpetuates an overarching unconscious or even a conscious bias from occupational therapists who don't have lived experience, resulting in ableism. This ableism then directly affects practice by increasing the likelihood of ableist experiences encountered among those we serve. More research needs to be carried out to address this cause and effect. I've heard too many stories of healthcare professionals putting people into boxes and not actually utilizing their therapeutic use of self to build up a relationship. We need people to enter the profession who have that lived experience so they can add authenticity and understanding to their practice. I'm not saying we need to be a profession full of disabled occupational therapists (even if my community does rock), because what we truly need is diversity to make sure that everyone is represented. How can the profession establish frameworks and make decisions without representing the general public? Collaboration and coproduction between service users and occupational therapists who have lived experienced themselves needs to be encouraged to look at these issues.

---

2   https://affinot.co.uk/ableotuk

I didn't have as much knowledge surrounding ableism back then as I do now. However, I think it was the final year of my degree when my belongingness to the course was at its highest since we then began unpicking the meaning of empowered practice. This wasn't covered in great depth within the course content – it was something that my peers and I co-created. Yes, it was great to have this opportunity and the module lead did essentially give us free rein to do what we wanted, but part of me was questioning why it had to come from those with lived experienced yet again rather than the higher education institution itself. By all means ask us and learn from us, but don't tokenize us. I chose what I wanted to share within those sessions, but I still felt that I had to place myself in a vulnerable position and share my trauma to make an impact. I'm used to sharing my own experiences in my talks, which can be repetitive and difficult, but most of the time I do it in front of audiences that don't know me, so it's fine. But sharing my ableist stories, particularly surrounding my experiences on placement, with my peers on that very course was daunting.

The sessions on 'empowered practice conversations' centred round language use and terminology, and covered a lot about oppression within the two-hour sessions. We all spoke about our experiences, considering them from an intersectional point of view. The conversations stemmed from a lot of ableist, racist and homophobic language that was used on the course and in practice. We couldn't believe, as individuals who would soon go out and work with these communities, that these offensive slurs were being used in lecture theatres. This language was and still is used so frequently in a professional setting, and it just has to stop – for example, the use of the phrase 'wheelchair-bound' rather than the preferred term 'wheelchair user'. Do I even need to explain that one? No one is bound by a wheelchair – a wheelchair can enable chronically ill people to have more energy and be in less pain. I could go on forever!

The sessions were very raw and this is why we named them 'conversations' and not 'workshops'. Another purpose of the sessions was to reiterate that everyone needs to continue learning and we must all listen and work together to improve. It was a safe space and it was endearing to see the conversations develop over the two-hour sessions as people shared their lived experiences – so much so that we even had different cohorts and professions joining our conversations. This resulted in **Millie Pollitt** and I presenting our reflections at the Occupational

Therapy and Physiotherapy Practice Educator Conference at our university (Pollitt and Vine 2021).

> The **Reflexivity in Practice Worksheet** (available in the Appendix) was written by Millie Pollitt (with a small contribution from myself). The reflective toolkit includes some important topics that I can't do justice to the way that Millie does!

I don't challenge practice just because I like to make waves but because I want to improve a profession that I'm so passionate about. Challenging this profession correctly not only enhances practice but also furthers our understanding of different communities. So why are we not making sure that the future generation of occupational therapists is fully equipped to do this? Simply because we are not recognizing our unique perspectives or standpoints that come from our experiences and social position. We therefore need to value this and create space within occupational therapy training to allow the creation of equity-based activities, sustaining more inclusive cultures and environments (Thomas 2022).

However, as we've established, adding new content into training isn't enough. We need to re-evaluate the content that students are currently being taught to ensure that they qualify as anti-discriminatory practitioners. Despite the fact that occupational therapists may know their role in addressing disablist structural barriers, they are less likely to go against the status quo and structural ableist ideology (Whalley Hammell 2022). This is because they need people with lived experience to point out the ableist privileges that are enjoyed by non-disabled occupational therapists themselves (Whalley Hammell 2022).

Occupational therapy training highlights tragedy through 'inspiration porn' (Grenier 2021, p.270). Isn't it funny how I came to this exact same conclusion in the first few chapters just through using my own experiences? It's about making students aware that these 'medical' areas of occupational therapy practices have ableist flaws. And not only they are ableist; these practices don't actually align with the core values of the profession in the first place. The medical model absolutely has its place as it allows for easy discharge of patients from medical services and will allow patients to qualify under insurance restrictions, depending on their location. As someone who's never worked in clinical practice, it would be wrong of me to judge without truly knowing the constraints and pressures of this fast-paced practice. But we need to make students aware of this to ensure that they not only become anti-ableist allies in practice, but also actually don't forget the core values of the profession.

There are also some views within occupational therapy theory itself that could be challenged – for example, activities of daily living (ADLs). ADLs are often broken down into self-care, productivity and leisure, and are taught as the main three domains of occupation (Creek *et al.* 2022). Some disabled people may be unable to work and 'be productive', but this should not be a measure of their social value (Whalley Hammell 2022), and these domains are also not applicable to all communities and all cultures. Too much emphasis is placed on 'independent self-care', and some disabled people may not be able to participate in this without carers (Whalley Hammell 2022, p.6). Furthermore, an unpaid carer may not be able to classify their caring responsibilities under these domains fully. By viewing self-care as 'independent' (not participated in with assistance), the occupational therapy profession is actively promoting the ideology that disabled people are 'unproductive' or 'dependent' (Whalley Hammell 2022, p.6). This is a neoliberalist viewpoint (Whalley Hammell 2022). There are a lot of things I can't do independently, such as making a meal, but I'm fine with that. Yes, I will never be able to cook a roast dinner independently, but that does not devalue my worth.

'Neoliberalism is based on the assumption that capitalism, the market, competition and the performance principle are the solution to close "justice gaps" within societies' (Gruber and Scherling 2020, cited in Schäfer 2019, p.49). Justice gaps are areas where marginalized groups have at least one unmet justice requirement or social inequity (World Justice Project 2019). Occupational therapy training enforces neoliberalism, with some disability theorists suggesting rehabilitative goals may be less about the individual's quality of life and more about social conformity (Whalley Hammell 2022). Is this view explicitly taught to healthcare students? These ableist concepts are either knowingly or unknowingly taught to students as the profession continues to do little to challenge established norms. We therefore need to be analysing occupational therapy models of practice, assessments and goal-setting processes through an anti-discriminatory lens, and look into the history of the profession to understand the grass roots of ableist injustices within the profession.

As we can see from the critical research and from my experiences, the profession creates quite a divide between occupational therapists and disabled people, therefore failing to acknowledge disabled occupational therapists themselves who cross over between these two categories (Whalley Hammell 2022). Occupational therapists are put on a pedestal, fostering a power imbalance between them and disabled people. Disabled professionals represent the people we serve and could even be students sitting in that very lecture theatre. So how must they feel when training refuses to acknowledge their existence? Admittedly, my own knowledge has increased through research but, as a disabled student, I certainly felt the anguish and lack of representation. This is why I've been asked to write this very book, to highlight that occupational therapists can be disabled and service users too!

Grenier (2021, p.271) calls for the 'radical dismantling and rebuilding of key professional frameworks and models to eliminate ableist disability discourses'. Grenier (2021) summarizes the research by saying that we need to be recruiting more students and academics with lived experience of disability. As someone who has been both a student and an academic, I completely agree with this proposition. I'm not 'blowing my own trumpet' here, but I don't think I was employed just because I 'tick that box' of diversity. I was employed because, using my lived experiences and my knowledge of being an activist, I am in an authentic position to question practice. For future disabled occupational therapists to return to academia, their degrees must be accessible in the first place and not perpetuate ableist experiences. Those of us with protected characteristics should be enrolled on to programmes and employed because we are needed and valued, not because we tick the inclusivity box!

The question is, can we facilitate change and rebuilding within these systems, or is it better to dismantle the existing systems and create new ones entirely? I hope that most occupational therapists reading this have, like me, accepted that the profession has injustices that need to be eliminated. My question, however, is, which solution addressing these injustices is the best use of our time, energy and resources?

Addressing systemic injustices takes time and action, and this chapter can't change existing processes on its own. We need to stop sugar-coating the profession; overall I've had some amazing experiences, but the profession has its flaws. Students not only need to be accommodated for, but we owe it to them to show the pitfalls of the profession too, so we can all work alongside each other to address the current inequities.

NOT SO TERRIBLE...P.A.L.S.Y. REFLECTIVE LOG
Pausing
Stop and think about what you have read in this chapter. What are your main takeaway points? What are your main questions?

....

....

....

Analysing
Why did this resonate with you?

....

....

....

Learning
What did you learn from this?

....

....

....

Solving
What actions need to be put into place?

....

....

....

Your plan

How will you achieve these actions? What are your goals?

. . . .

. . . .

. . . .

References

Atwal, A., Sriram, V. and McKay, E., for BAME OT (2021) 'Making a difference: Belonging, diversity and inclusion in occupational therapy.' *British Journal of Occupational Therapy 84*, 11, 671–672. Accessed on 16 June 2023 at https://doi. org/10.1177/03080226211031797

Brentnall, C. and Stanbury, D. (2023) 'Compassion and Cooperation for Graduate Attributes.' University of Huddersfield, 23 February.

Creek, J., Bryant, W., Fieldhouse, J. and Bannigan, K. (2022) *Creek's Occupational Therapy and Mental Health* (6th edn). Glasgow: Elsevier.

Dobson Waters, S. and Torgerson, C.J. (2021) 'Dyslexia in higher education: A systematic review of interventions used to promote learning.' *Journal of Further and Higher Education 45*, 2, 226–256. Accessed on 16 June 2023 at https://doi.org/10.1080/03 09877X.2020.1744545

Falzon, R. (2021) 'Dyslexia and Academic Life.' In J. Glazzard and S. Stones (eds) *Dyslexia*. IntechOpen. Accessed on 16 June 2023 at www.intechopen.com/chapters/74094

Graham, M., Bacha, S., Martinez, E. and Vine, G. (2022) 'Feeling Connected: Exploring Equity, Diversity and Belonging with Undergraduate Occupational Therapy Students.' Paper Presentation. Royal College of Occupational Therapists 45th Annual Virtual Conference, June.

Grenier, M. (2021) 'Patient cases formulations and oppressive disability discourses in occupational therapy education.' *Canadian Journal of Occupational Therapy 88*, 3, 266–272. Accessed on 1 January 2023 at https://doi.org/10.1177/0008417421005882

Gruber, B. and Scherling, G. (2020) 'The relevance of unmasking neoliberal narratives for a decolonized human rights and peace education.' *International Journal of Human Rights Education 4*, 1. Accessed on 1 January 2023 at https://repository. usfca.edu/ijhre/vol4/iss1/3

Hortop, A. (2022) 'Time to Change the Occupational Therapy Blue Print, Embracing the New Architecture of Belonging-Centred Practice.' Paper. Royal College of Occupational Therapists 45th Annual Virtual Conference, 15 June.

Iwama, M.K. (2006) 'The Kawa (River) Model: Client-Centred Rehabilitation in Cultural Context.' In S. Davis (ed.) *Rehabilitation: The Use of Theories and Models in Practice* (pp.147–168). Edinburgh: Churchill Livingstone Elsevier.

Malfitano, A.P.S., Whiteford, G. and Molineux, M. (2019) 'Transcending the individual: The promise and potential of collectivist approaches in occupational therapy.' *Scandinavian Journal of Occupational Therapy 28*, 3, 188–200. Accessed on 17 February 2023 at https://doi.org/10.1080/11038128.2019.1693627

Murphy, A. and Stevenson, J. (2018) 'Occupational potential and possible selves of master's level healthcare students with dyslexia: A narrative inquiry.' *Journal of Occupational Science 26*, 1, 18–28.

NHS (National Health Service) (2019) 'Chapter 2: More NHS action on prevention and health inequalities.' In *Online Version of the NHS Long Term Plan*. Accessed on 20 December 2022 at www.longtermplan.nhs.uk/online-version/chapter-2-more-nhs-action-on-prevention-and-health-inequalities

Pedler, M.E., Willis, R. and Nieuwoudt, J.E. (2021) 'A sense of belonging at university: Student retention, motivation and enjoyment.' *Journal of Further and Higher Education 46*, 3, 397–408. Accessed on 20 December 2022 at https://doi.org/10.10 80/0309877X.2021.1955844

Pillow, D.R., Malone, G.P. and Hale, W.J. (2015) 'The need to belong and its association with fully satisfying relationships: A tale of two measures.' *Personality and Individual Differences 74*, 259–264. Accessed on 5 January 2023 at https://doi.org/10.1016/j.paid.2014.10.031

Pino, M. and Mortari, L. (2014) 'The inclusion of students with dyslexia in higher education: A systematic review using narrative synthesis.' *Dyslexia 20*, 4, 346–369. Accessed on 16 June 2023 at https://onlinelibrary.wiley.com/doi/10.1002/dys.1484

Pollitt, M. and Vine, G. (2021) *Empowered Practice Conversations: Practice Educator Edition*. Occupational Therapy and Physiotherapy Practice Educator Conference, 23 June, Sheffield Hallam University.

Pywell, S. (2021) 'The reasonable adjustment/request of dealing in to education: Being an anti-ableist educator in face-to-face classrooms.' *Centre for Collaborative Learning* [Blog], 21 October, University of Central Lancashire (UCLan). Accessed on 10 December 2022 at https://ccl.uclan.ac.uk/2021/10/21/the-reasonable-adjustment-request-of-dialing-in-to-education-being-an-anti-ableist-educator-in-face-to-face-classrooms

Schäfer, A. (2019) *Die Alternativlosigkeit von Bildung: Zur Dialektik der Bildung in Neoliberalismus*. Weinheim: Beltz Juventa.

Thomas, D.S.P. (2022) 'Belonging matters.' *AdvanceHE*, 11 October. Accessed on 20 December 2022 at www.advance-he.ac.uk/news-and-views/belonging-matters

Werdelin Education (2019) 'Cooperative learning defined: Easy. Efficient. Inexpensive.' Accessed on 15 March 2023 at https://werdelin.co.uk/triple-welcome/cldefined

WFOT (World Federation of Occupational Therapists) (2016) *Minimum Standards for the Education of Occupational Therapists*. Accessed on 7 April 2023 at www.wfot.org/resources/new-minimum-standards-for-the-education-of-occupational-therapists-2016-e-copy

Whalley Hammell, K. (2014) 'Belonging, occupation, and human well-being: An exploration' ['Appurtenance, occupation et bien-être humain: Une étude exploratoire']. *Canadian Journal of Occupational Therapy 81*, 1, 39–50. Accessed on 1 January 2023 at https://doi.org/10.1177/0008417413520489

Whalley Hammell, K. (2022) 'A call to resist occupational therapy's promotion of ableism.' *Scandinavian Journal of Occupational Therapy*. Accessed on 1 January 2023 at https://doi.org/10.1080/11038128.2022.2130821

World Justice Project (2019) *Measuring the Justice Gap*. Accessed on 5 January 2023 at https://worldjusticeproject.org/our-work/publications/special-reports/measuring-justice-gap

PART THREE

My Early Career Experiences

CHAPTER NINE

Becoming a Registered Occupational Therapist

I am not sorry that I am disabled, and nor should anyone else be.

Telling my story about becoming a registered occupational therapist was never my intention when I started putting my book proposal together, never mind dedicating a whole chapter to that part of my life! But when I was first contacted to write a book proposal, I was asked to write about disabled activism within the occupational therapy profession, so this chapter became an essential inclusion I needed to share with everyone.

You cannot call yourself an occupational therapist, or practice as an occupational therapist, until you are registered with the Health & Care Professions Council (HCPC)[1] if you live in the UK, or CORU – Regulating Health and Social Care Professionals[2] if you live in Ireland. So the moment I received confirmation of my degree classification, I downloaded the online application form and started to collate all the information I needed. I had attended a seminar at university that explained the application process, so I felt fairly confident about filling out the form. However, as a disabled occupational therapy student, I knew that the 'Fitness to Practise' section of the form would take a lot of time and effort to fill out in detail, unlike the brief forms for my non-disabled university friends. I have been disabled all my life so I'm pretty used to intensive form-filling, and feel I can be accurate about my own needs without too much stress.

The 'Fitness to Practise' section, however, wasn't exactly what I was

---

1   www.hcpc-uk.org/registration/getting-on-the-register/uk-applications/uk-application-forms
2   www.coru.ie

expecting, and was an overall confusing experience! In fact, what I had anticipated as a whole section of text was just one 'yes/no' question. This asked me if I 'had any physical or mental health conditions that would impair my fitness to practise'. Of course, this resulted in a lot of internal debate on my part.

Yes, I do have a condition that affects the way I practise, but does it affect my fitness to practise? Yes, my disability *could* affect that way I work with others in practice but, on the other hand, in a properly supported and adapted environment, I can work just as efficiently as any other non-disabled occupational therapist. Yes, my disability *could* affect the way I communicate with others through barriers such as speech clarity, but if I communicate using AAC via text-to-speech, or utilize technology to email those I work with, then there are no barriers here either. Do you see how 'yes/no' questions and the use of 'would' doesn't help define my disability and my *true* access needs with cerebral palsy? *Would appears unequivocal whereas the word could is much more accessible. Health fluctuates and no two years with a disability, or days, for that matter, are the same.*

So do I need to tick 'yes', my disability does affect the way I practise? After a discussion with my parents, we decided that ticking 'yes' would be the best course of action. I ticked that box, knowing that I would need reasonable adjustments to be made under the Equality Act 2010[3] for me to practise. My placement experiences had taught me that in order to be a skilled and effective occupational therapist, and to use my training to its full capacity, I would need support and modifications. I knew that ticking this box would come with a bit of red tape and delay, but it had to be done, and it had to be done correctly. The decision to *positively* disclose my disability was made to ensure the safety of those I would be working with in practice.

Box ticked, the form was sent to the administrations office at the HCPC. About three weeks later I received a response. Although I hadn't wholly expected to be registered on the 'first try' since I had ticked that box, and had expected an automatic response saying that the HCPC would need more information on my health, I definitely hadn't banked on receiving the actual email I received.

The email informed me that they were '*sorry to hear that I have a health condition that could impair my fitness to practise*'. They also said

---

3   www.legislation.gov.uk/ukpga/2010/15/contents

that I had not provided any evidence about how my condition affected me, and I needed to provide some. I understand that some people reading this may not be as familiar with disability language and terminology as others, but 'sorry to hear' is not okay. Coming from a nationwide, well-renowned council like the HCPC, especially one as centred in healthcare, they should have been more sensitive in their wording. By saying they were 'sorry to hear' about my health condition they were evoking pity; I felt that they were almost commiserating with me on my disability, suggesting that my health condition was more of a negative thing that people should be 'sorry' for me for having.

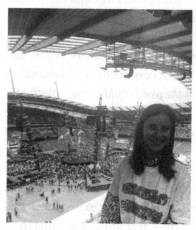

Image 9.1. *Georgia, a white female, at a concert, stood to the right, high up in the stands, with the concert stage behind her. She is wearing a top with two parallel horizontal lines covered in a paint splatter pattern over an animal print blouse.*

Now obviously these things are not explicit, but words matter, and how you speak *about* key subjects and people is just as important as how you speak *to* them. It is the 21st century and disability is not a bad thing, or a bad word, for that matter.

I personally found the phrase very ableist. I am not sorry that I am disabled, and nor should anyone else be. I know that I am disability confident and this confidence has fuelled my disability activism and me generally being vocal about disability rights. When I applied to study occupational therapy in 2017, I was fully aware that I would have limitations within practice.

Having this forewarning of my limitations allowed me to have plenty of time to comprehend that the way I practise will look different to how others practise. Although I know that my practice will be different to a non-disabled occupational therapist, I felt that the reply from the HCPC to my application was belittling, implying that I did not have a good understanding of my own needs. Let's just say, I did not feel like an 'expert by experience' in this instance. The email also implied that it was my fault that I had not given any evidence of my disability. I had read both the form and the guide to filling out the registration form thoroughly, and there was no mention of how I should provide evidence of my disability. As you can imagine, I found the email wholly frustrating, and it was really quite upsetting feeling so misunderstood. Despite my frustration I still had to get on the register in order to legally practise as an occupational therapist in the UK. I had spent three years to pass all of my placements and gain a first class honours degree, so I didn't want to waste all of this time and passion.

At this point, I had two weeks to get back to the email with my 'evidence' so it was on my mind a lot. But what evidence was I supposed to give? I have provided evidence of my disability multiple times over the years so I am not fazed by that, but the question of how I *think* my disability will affect my practice is not straightforward, so the evidence I needed to send off was harder to pinpoint. At this time, I had yet to have a job offer and did not know what environment I would be working in. The occupational therapy profession is so diverse it's very hard to create a generic picture of my overarching needs in every single environment an occupational therapist could work in. And in this vicious circle, I couldn't apply for jobs because I wasn't registered with the HCPC.

I found myself in quite a predicament, so I decided to reach out to some of my friends and colleagues for advice. As a founding member of AbleOTUK,[4] I had formed a close bond with the others and I reached out to them for advice. I had rung the HCPC after receiving the email, asking for advice on which evidence pieces to provide, and the adviser on the phone had replied, 'Whatever you think.' I didn't find this helpful as it didn't narrow the really wide scope of the huge pile of 21 years' worth of medical letters and university placement assessments that I had in front of me!

The support from AbleOTUK was gratefully received during this time, and knowing that I could talk to others with similar experiences

---

4   https://affinot.co.uk/ableotuk

certainly helped. As a group, we also felt we desperately needed to address the ableism within the applications process. Due to AbleOTUK being a new network at the time, my current issues just highlighted another area of practice that our group needed to address. My experiences sparked new ideas within the group, fuelled by the anger of those who were qualified and who had experienced similar issues. There were also student members in the group who still had their HCPC application ahead of them. Retelling my experience fuelled some anxiousness and uncertainty for them as their worries about registering with the HCPC had suddenly amplified after knowing about my issues. I did regret this knock-on effect, and if anything, that was what spurred me on. My intention was to ensure that no future graduate would experience the feeling I had felt when reading that email.

AbleOTUK gave me loads of information and I felt very supported; we collated information from the HCPC and Royal College of Occupational Therapists (RCOT), so we had everything we thought we needed and read through the HCPC examples they'd given. Reading through the examples, however, highlighted an even split between healthcare professionals who had specifically named their health conditions and those who had not.

If you're in a similar situation, the **HCPC booklet** 'Health, disability and becoming a health and care professional' might help your understanding, even though it isn't perfect (HCPC 2015).

The booklet certainly has its flaws, it is missing information and it needs updating, but it might go some way to helping your understanding. The best thing to come from reading it was that it reassured me that I did not need to give the HCPC pages of information on my cerebral palsy. I also feel hopeful as I know that the HCPC is now doing a lot of work to further enhance its equality, diversity and belonging strategy (HCPC 2022).

Here, though, I was stuck again with a huge dilemma – did I need to specifically disclose my cerebral palsy, or just the specific effects it would have on my practice? After multiple discussions with members from AbleOTUK, I also got in touch with my university lecturers, and they were not happy about my situation. They advised me to revisit my pre-placement learning agreement, and this was a very helpful suggestion as I could detail the adjustments I had needed on placement and would therefore need in practice. I did know some of the adjustments I needed, but would a vague picture be enough for the HCPC?

Time to send the email. In the end, I did disclose my cerebral palsy as I had already been waiting long enough and really didn't want to slow the process down further since I personally had no objection to the HCPC knowing about my disability. I know I do not owe anyone my medical history, but I am very passionate about this profession, and I wanted to ensure that I did everything I could to provide the utmost care and respect to those I would be working with.

> To find out more about what you need to disclose to the HCPC and what you don't, read 'Health and character declarations – our experience' (Keen and Vine 2023).

Unfortunately, the next stage of the process was no easier and it involved a lot of my time chasing things up. It was a busy time of year for the HCPC, who had lots of applications from newly qualified healthcare professionals to process.[5] However, knowing that I could have been on the register for over a month and allowed to apply for jobs was frustrating. I had seen a few potential jobs that I had wanted to apply for, one of which was online and seemed very accessible for me. But I could not apply, as I was told I had to be registered, even when I emailed to explain about my situation.

Although you can work as an occupational therapy assistant until your registration has come through, with so much uncertainty around my registration, it wasn't looking promising. At this point, I decided that I really wanted to get into the workplace and made the move to start applications for openings for occupational therapy assistants. This was pretty disheartening after studying for three years at university and working so hard to get my degree alongside managing my disability. I

---

5   www.hcpc-uk.org/registration/getting-on-the-register/uk-applications/uk-application-forms

still had my fingers crossed that the HCPC would return my registration sooner than we were all thinking.

During this time, I got in touch with the RCOT. I was already having a planned meeting with the new Chief Executive, Steve Ford, before everything with the HCPC had happened, and so I mentioned my struggles in passing, as it was, understandably, occupying much of my thoughts at the time. The support of the RCOT during this time definitely didn't go unnoticed; I was, and still am, so grateful that Steve acted straight away and put me in touch with the Professional Advisory Team to help me deal with the whole situation. By then it was becoming evident that this unexpected battle to get on the register was affecting my mental health.

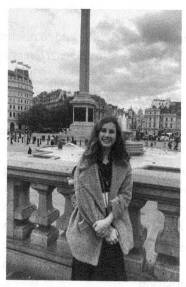

Image 9.2. *Georgia, a white female, in Trafalgar Square after going to the Royal College of Occupational Therapists Awards ceremony. She is wearing a dress and a fluffy coat, with a backpack on.*

I thought that I had done the hard part by completing my degree! Between not finding a job and not yet being able to call myself an occupational therapist, I was massively doubting my abilities. My internalized ableism had also been heightened by all the external ableism I was facing going through this process. I had just spent three years, working hard at my degree, and now I may not be able to practise?

Speaking to the Professional Advisory Team helped me to refocus, and they reassured me that I was entering the right profession. They also reminded me that I had disclosed my disability positively, and this gave me the boost I needed. This red tape was not going to stop me in my tracks, so why would I let mental fatigue with the situation stop me? I needed to keep working on this problem, and emailing them was getting me nowhere.

So I picked up the phone, which is another anxiety-provoking experience for me due to my speech impairment, but after days of trying I got through to an HCPC adviser, and luckily my dad was around to ensure that I was not misunderstood. From the phone call, I learned that I now had a case manager who was reviewing the evidence and details within my case.

Yet more radio silence occurred, and another three weeks went by before more contact was made and, once again, this contact was initiated by me. It was a very long, drawn-out and exhausting process. I finally got an email informing me that my supporting information regarding my fitness to practise had been accepted and I would soon be registered! At long last!

I was thrilled that this process was coming to a close and so relieved that I now had more opportunities when looking for jobs, although the end of the email reminded me that I could not yet call myself an occupational therapist (my registration came through days later, though, so I didn't have another long wait, thankfully). After waiting for three months and going through such a challenging time with the registration process, that reminder did feel like a bit of a kick in the teeth, but at least the gruelling part of the process was finally finished!

I understood that my registration was never going to be straightforward, but I was not expecting my mental health to be impacted this much. Again, this news could have been given to me quite differently, and even though now I could see the light at the end of the tunnel, the process was not as smooth as it could have so easily been. The whole registration process is ableist as it puts disabled graduates at a disadvantage to non-disabled graduates. This just should not happen. Entering the profession after studying should be the most exciting time in your career, not filled with so much uncertainty.

A few weeks after registering I was vocal about my story on social media and my website, which was hard. I did not want to be seen as 'bad mouthing' the HCPC and therefore get kicked off the register, especially after it had taken me so long to get on it. But I had to raise awareness, and it was actually the RCOT themselves, AbleOTUK and my supervisor, Margaret, who pushed me to do so.

In a meeting with the RCOT and AbleOTUK, we discussed my issues with the registration process and the RCOT themselves said how I needed to be more vocal about this, as well as offering to raise my issues anonymously with the HCPC themselves – although I think by the time that the RCOT had actually raised my issues, the HCPC may have had a sneaky suspicion as to who these frustrations were about.

Immediately after the meeting with the RCOT I decided to email Margaret to ask her if I should tell my story on my blog. I knew it would be a bold move, yet I felt that it had to be done. The registration process was not going to improve without a noise being made. To my relief, Margaret replied with the go-ahead. Many people in the occupational therapy community on Twitter were following my story and knew that I was having a hard time finding a job. I know they knew something else was happening because I had tweeted about *finally* being on the register, so I guess now was my time to tell my story and highlight the issues.

I wrote the blog much like I've written this chapter – in frustration – and it felt amazing to finally get that frustration out on paper. I was still cautious and kept writing 'the register' instead of the HCPC. Yet the edited blog I received back from Margaret was a bit of a shock as she suggested that I actually name the HCPC. I was apprehensive for this level of exposure against a big council, despite them doing wrong, but my blog went live anyway.

The blog made noise all right, and was my most viewed blog post of 2021 and still made it in my top three most viewed posts in 2022. The occupational therapy community once again sent so much support and kindness my way, and it was greatly appreciated. I was still nervous, but everyone's support made it all worthwhile and made me so pleased that I had told my story. Everyone kept tagging the HCPC in their comments; the register heard thanks to everyone's support, and I got my point across.

My point was heard: victory, right? Not really – the real victory is in seeing the end result. Now the HCPC knew my story, they had to act on it.

I have now learned from speaking to previous lecturers and from exploring the ins and outs of the situation that my disability never affected my fitness to practise as I passed all my placements. This is because any reasonable adjustments I would need would be put into place between myself and my workplace and not the HCPC. Universities need to put processes in place to clarify this for future students with disabilities; if this had been in place when I qualified I may have not ticked the 'yes' box, and none of the above would have happened.

I still have the worry of being penalized for falsehoods or incorrectly ticking the 'no' box. This is an ethical and moral dilemma that needs examining, and clearer guidance is required from the HCPC. Positive disclosure should be encouraged for those who want to disclose and for those who need to disclose when thinking about any fitness to practise challenges further on in their careers.

Systems should be put into place so that disabled healthcare students or those with a long-term health condition have access to the correct support to be able to register with the HCPC. As well as working with the HCPC to improve this fitness to practise process, I understand that registration cannot be granted until qualifications are confirmed. However, disabled students may be penalized in their ability to apply for jobs if their forms take longer to be approved, and they won't then be HCPC registered until later than a non-disabled student. Disabled students should be given an ability to begin the 'Fitness to Practise' section approval process before the end of the course so that they are not disadvantaged and left facing an agonizing wait once qualified.

Well, what if disclosure is needed? Although the article signposted above should help with this and answer some of the commonly asked questions and address any misconceptions, I am pleased that after I approached them, I am now working directly with the HCPC to change the registration process. They have already changed the registration question to 'Do you have any physical or mental health condition which may affect your ability to practise safely and effectively in the profession to which your application relates?' Along with the team at AbleOTUK, I will do everything I can to ensure that no healthcare graduate experiences the same problems as I did. This journey with the HCPC was incredibly challenging, yet it ignited new passions within me to improve this process for others, and I'm pleased to report that we are making progress.

As a student, I was concerned about being a disabled activist in this profession. I always thought that qualifying as an occupational therapist would mean leaving my disabled activist roots behind due to working within professional guidelines, imposed by the HCPC themselves. Yet the experience I had has made me realize how much I can and will use my disabled activist skills to challenge ableism within the profession in the hope that justice can be achieved.

Good luck with your journey towards registering; I hope that it is a lot more straightforward than mine!

NOT SO TERRIBLE...P.A.L.S.Y. REFLECTIVE LOG

Pausing
Stop and think about what you have read in this chapter. What are your main takeaway points? What are your main questions?

....

....

....

Analysing
Why did this resonate with you?

....

....

....

Learning
What did you learn from this?

....

....

....

Solving

What actions need to be put into place?

. . . .

. . . .

. . . .

Your plan

How will you achieve these actions? What are your goals?

. . . .

. . . .

. . . .

References

HCPC (Health & Care Professions Council) (2015) 'Health, disability and becoming a health and care professional' [Booklet]. London: HCPC. Accessed on 17 February 2022 at www.hcpc-uk.org/students/health-disability-and-becoming-a-health-and-care-professional

HCPC (2022) 'Our commitment to equality, diversity and inclusion.' Accessed on 10 April 2023 at www.hcpc-uk.org/about-us/work-for-us/become-a-partner/our-commitment-to-equality-diversity-and-inclusion

Keen, A. and Vine, G. (2023) 'Health and character declarations – our experience.' OTnews, May, 54–55.

CHAPTER TEN

The Accessible Job Hunt

News flash! Not every Band 5 occupational therapist is a young, non-disabled person, or any band or grade for that matter!

In the months leading up to finishing university I began looking for my first occupational therapy post. I started looking early for multiple reasons; first, because I knew that it was going to take me longer to ensure my access requirements were met, and second, because my work style in general thrives in structured, planned situations. Not knowing what I was going to be doing on finishing university did not sit well with me.

Throughout my life I have had structure, and due to my disability, many life events have been planned to the max. Therefore, my goal was to secure my first role before I finished university, so I started looking at jobs six months before qualifying. Unfortunately for me it didn't happen, and this caused implications for my mental health and internalized ableism as well as depleting my energy due to juggling job hunting as well as trying to get through the pressures of a final year degree course.

In fact, I was six months post-qualifying (so a year of job hunting in total) before I found my first job as a clinical demonstrator in occupational therapy at the University of Huddersfield. Finding this job was really a case of being in the right place at the right time. I know what you're thinking – that I must have gone through so many job interviews within that year. In actuality, I can count the amount of interviews that I attended on one hand. I personally found that getting through the interview stage was the easiest part (and even this was not truly 'easy'!). Finding a job that was suitable for my access needs was, in fact, the biggest challenge due to a lot of ableism.

I attended an interview for a role in a paediatric service and felt wholly undermined throughout the interview experience. The interviewers dismissed all of my various work experiences and qualifications and placed me in a stereotypical box because of my disability. I definitely felt that they were not prepared to make reasonable adjustments for my cerebral palsy. Nor were they prepared for me to challenge practice. I remember talking about adding a relatable, human approach, and how I could utilize my therapeutic use of self and experience of my own disability, when used appropriately, of course, but it still did not get a good response – like, seriously? I didn't get that job because my question at the end about continuing professional development opportunities was 'too vague' – of course a question about me wanting to enhance my skills personally and professionally wasn't good enough... I think we all know the real reason. We need a workforce that represents the communities we serve (NHS 2019), and this is before we tackle the internal systemic ableism! I most definitely would not have enjoyed working in that environment, and would have hugely disliked working with those in the professional world who see only my disability rather than my whole person skillset.

I do think my challenge would have been greater if I had gone for an occupational therapy role in perhaps a hospital setting; I might even be still searching for this inclusive accessible role! Unfortunately, providing reasonable adjustments isn't always easy, depending on the role, and this leads me on to my first spiel of this chapter: area of practice.

Choosing an area of practice is a minefield for any occupational therapist due to how vast the profession is, but selecting the right area of practice when you have a disability is even trickier! My advice would be to explore different areas of practice *within reason*; it would have been naive of me to think I could have just worked in any occupational therapy role, anywhere. Many newly qualified occupational therapists start on rotation. This is where you literally rotate between different areas in that setting (such as different wards or departments in a hospital or even across a trust). In general, this gives newly qualified occupational therapists a glimpse of the variation of job roles. However, trying to ensure that each of these different locations, roles and team dynamics were suitable for my access needs would be really complicated! A hospital rotation would have been particularly complex as I certainly wouldn't have been able to work on a ward, and neither do I want to. I could have gone for these jobs to 'have a try', but with the knowledge that any new movement, role or non-adapted occupation could cause me increased pain and fatigue, this wouldn't be something that I would enjoy.

This doesn't mean that we can't explore our options; after all, you don't know unless you try. If you are interested in a particular area of practice but you are unsure whether this would suit you and your access needs, then contact the organization for more information. Ask to do some shadowing for a short period to get a feel of whether the role is suitable for you, and also enjoyable. I know how deflating this can feel when you've worked so hard to finally be fully qualified or you've acquired a disability after being in the field a while and you do deserve that post, but having a short-term trial period in this new area of practice (if you can afford to) would definitely be beneficial in the long run.

When I was still searching for a job for six months after qualifying it really affected my mental health – especially when most of my peers had a job lined up on finishing university. But looking back it gave me the chance to partake in so many opportunities I wouldn't have had time for if I'd gone straight into work. I worked on my blog *Not So Terrible Palsy*,[1] represented charities close to my heart through being promoted to head ambassador at CP Teens UK,[2] and got to grow in confidence while speaking at conferences.

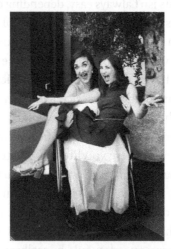

Image 10.1. *Two white females. Georgia is sat on her friend Georgina's knee, and Georgina is in her manual wheelchair. They are making goofy expressions and are all dolled up for the CP Teens UK Charity Ball.*

---

1   https://notsoterriblepalsy.com
2   www.cpteensuk.org

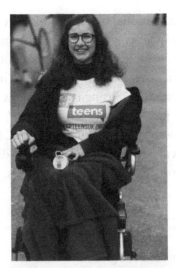

Image 10.2. *Georgia, a white female, in her electric wheelchair wearing a CP Teens UK t-shirt.*

Of course I had an urge to dive straight into work, just like any other newly qualified professional, as I wanted to gain clinical skills and knowledge. I was feeling that I was starting to lack confidence and had huge imposter syndrome when thinking about traditional roles, never mind anything else. I felt out of my depth, undeserving and under-qualified for the roles that I had applied for, despite having just as much passion, experience and as many qualifications as any other new professional. So why does going for a traditional role versus a non-clinical or slightly non-traditional role depend on experience? It took me a long time to be okay with the fact that I didn't get the clinical role post-qualifying that I was longing for and had built up in my mind. I have now realized that I was never going to fully enjoy and thrive in any other role; my previous academic adviser helped me realize that I had a different skillset than those who do prosper in these areas, but that there were so many other roles and roles yet to be found in the hugely diverse world of occupational therapy!

Throughout my studies, I was never a traditional student, as you have probably gathered by now, so why would I want to be a traditional practitioner? Yes, my disability limits the areas of practice I can work in, but my student experiences enable me to utilize skills that not many occupational therapists have, so I definitely shouldn't ignore this integral part of my personal and professional identity. Aside from that, what is a 'traditional job' in occupational therapy speak anyway? For a long time I called my first post-qualifying role 'non-traditional', and even wrote a lot of content about my role using this phrase, but it's not 'non-traditional' at all – a lot of occupational therapists work in academia. I'm still an occupational therapist and using my core skills as an occupational therapist daily in my job; just because it's not the 'gold standard' route for a new graduate doesn't make it 'non-traditional'. I have since learned to be more confident about utilizing my skills as a disabled person, and this confidence is through connecting with others.

TOP TIP

✓ Use your connections and groups.

I know as a co-founder I am biased, but I found AbleOTUK's peer support group particularly helpful as we are all experiencing or have experienced similar challenges. It's great to be able to talk to disabled peers and see if they have found ways to overcome a particular challenge that seems insurmountable for you at the moment. If you're interested in a particular role, speak to other occupational therapists with disabilities about their experiences so you have all the information to make an informed decision. Remember – if this is your first role, most occupational therapists don't find their dream job initially, and you are not alone! No matter what area your 'for now' role is, it's all experience to enhance your personal and professional development.

Now we come on to our favourite topic – you guessed it...disclosure. To disclose or not to disclose, it's that simple, right?

We all know that's not the case, and when it comes to disclosure in the workplace, it can quite complex, and this is why I like to talk about it right from the start of the job hunting process. Whether it's disclosing on the application form or disclosing at occupational health, the turmoil of disclosure creeps in. Unfortunately, as you read before with my paediatric interview, you can (entirely wrongly) be seen as having reduced abilities if you have a disability, due to ableism within recruitment teams. Some people decide not to disclose their health conditions at all, which, believe you me, can at times feel like the best option.

Personally, I disclose during the application process and always tick that box, which almost guarantees me an interview under the Disability Confident employer scheme (DWP 2021). This encourages employers to take action to improve the recruitment, retainment and development of disabled people. The first time I ticked the box, to almost guarantee me an interview, I felt so guilty. But why? Why, yet again, should I let my internalized ableism take over and why should I feel guilty about ticking a box that I am fully entitled to tick?

After spending so long on my application I wanted to make sure that my application was put to good use. Due to my disability I have a smaller pot of energy compared to a non-disabled person, and some days that pot of energy is very small, meaning that tasks can be made a lot harder and take a lot longer. Therefore it can be heart-breaking when I find that my energy and effort on a specific task wasn't worth it, but ticking that box almost guarantees that my energy has been put to some good use! Ticking that box does not require a medical history, which makes a change as everything else has to be justified. Of course this is completely personal, but I just thought that I would point it out.

Most of the time I disclosed my cerebral palsy before applying for the job to save energy. I would ask about the day-to-day roles of the job to make sure that it was right for me (not forgetting that even if it was evidently not suitable, that reasonable adjustments should be put into place). At times this really helped. I've even been asked to go to the workplace and have a chat to find out more about the role – at the time I was really impressed after having had some rather ableist experiences in this process. This system with an in-person informal assessment and chat should be put into place for disabled employees everywhere, as it helps both the employer and potential employee work out if they are a good fit. As occupational therapists we know how much the environment impacts occupational performance (Duncan 2021), and nobody can truly understand what reasonable adjustments they need without knowing the environment in person!

Unfortunately, some of the pre-interview meetings really didn't help my overall experience. One time, I specifically mentioned that making adjustments to an individual wheelchair was very difficult for me. Imagine my surprise when I found that the interview practical assessment was exactly that one task: adjustment of a wheelchair! This was a really difficult situation for me as the practicalities of this action are very hard for my cerebral palsy without reasonable adjustments, so I was unsure if this was an intentional test to see if I could actually perform the task, or if they were testing me to check I could suitably ask for help when I needed it. Either way, when I defined my needs to them, they completely ignored my own advocacy and needs during their interview process – what was the point of the conversation about adjustments if they were just going to ignore everything I said?

There have also been times that disclosing via email has not worked out in my favour, and I have had replies back saying that I'd be 'too vulnerable' (the exact words about one position) in this environment. When I sent the email I did want honesty as, like I said, it helps me decide if I need to put my energy elsewhere and apply for other roles, but being described as 'too vulnerable' just in an email conversation is not right, and those professionals should definitely know that this is ableist. As occupational therapists we are taught to adapt the environment for those we serve, so why can't we do the same for those we work with? Surely going into a role where you are supervised by an occupational therapist you would have thought your potential manager would have a great skillset to help with adaptations and to make these kinds of decisions?

Something that I would do differently now is specifically ask what reasonable adjustments could be made for anything I specified as needing to be adjusted within that physical setting or role itself. Sometimes I'd quickly rule out the job just from that one email response. For example, being called 'too vulnerable' is an ableist response, and I would not want a person like that as my senior colleague and to work in that environment anyway. However, in other situations I should have asked more specific questions and used job-specific examples, asking things like: 'You've said that the role involves adjusting wheelchairs – I'd personally struggle with this some days, so could alternative interactions be put into place such as me telling someone how to adjust the wheelchair?' If you don't ask, you never know! I also think that getting these questions out of the way beforehand makes the interview process feel a lot easier.

I disclose my disability to my potential employer partly because this is so visible, and I have to address my speech impairment because I want to disclose my disability *positively*. Yes, it does pose some difficulties in practice, but I am fine with this. I know my strengths and weaknesses, as we all have them, disability or not. I'm a big fan of positive disclosure, and believe that a safe environment must be created to enhance positive disclosure so a person's access needs can be addressed, enabling them to thrive in the workplace using their disability as a tool.

Writing this down as a recommendation for other people makes the whole disclosure and adaptations process seem a lot easier than it actually is. We know that the psychological aspects of disclosing are tough, and it is, in fact, the hardest part of disclosing, but what makes this harder still is the fact that it doesn't get recognized. The fear of rejection creeps in – will they accept me? Will they believe me? Now I know I'm not best placed to be leading this discussion, as many aspects of my disability are visible to others, but those with invisible disabilities can often have amplified fears of people invalidating their needs. Disabled people must feel safe when disclosing, and safe spaces must be made to encourage positive disclosure. I think that until this is recognized and understood, some people will still feel uncomfortable in stating their needs, particularly if they are not visible.

My cerebral palsy is a very visible disability, but I can relate to this fear and anxiety as there are many parts of my disability that are hidden. On placement I really struggled with this and feared that the reasonable adjustments I needed were, in fact, unreasonable. The fact that this entered my mind demonstrates how heightened my internalized ableism was. These fears about advocating for reasonable adjustments are unfortunately well known in the disability community due to our own and others' previous life experiences. And not forgetting that internalized ableism 'would not exist without the real external oppression that forms the social climate in which we exist' (Marks 1999, cited in Kumari Campbell 2009, p.25). Therefore until this social climate's incorrect perceptions of those with disabilities is put right, disabled people will always have this fear.

Surely it should be occupational therapists who understand the importance of productivity and occupational belongingness to help promote positive disclosure in the workplace, and we can, by shifting our attitudes. Disclosure isn't a bad thing, and when done correctly and positively it can open up so many doors! I know you would want to be an approachable manager and a Disability Confident employer, so these changes need to be made. Employment and interviewing for new jobs are major milestones in a disabled person's life that *must* be dealt with correctly. Remember that saying you are a Disability Confident employer and actually being a Disability Confident employer are two different things.

> Visit the **Disability Confident employer scheme** to find out more about it and how to become an accessible employer (DWP 2021).

Stating that you 'consider yourself to have a disability' during the application process means that an interview offer should come with a section that asks if any adaptations need to be made to make the interview process easier. If this isn't the case, make sure you email your potential employer to state your access requirements for the interview. Before filling in this adaptation section make sure to read the email thoroughly and think about what's expected of you at that particular interview, including any practical tasks that you might be expected to complete.

For these physical elements, don't be afraid to ask what the specific task is, as you can then understand if you're going to need support or not. This has happened to me a few times, and I wish I had asked about this to save my energy overall. Of course, if you feel like you can do this independently, then go ahead and smash that interview, as sometimes it is certainly worth pushing ourselves. But if this is not doable without support, it doesn't make you any less of a fabulous potential employee! You should also think about what other support is needed, for example if you're asked to do a presentation at interview. Don't be afraid to make your adaptations known. I was worried about a particular online interview where I would be using my text-to-speech AAC to give a presentation; when I emailed the recruitment team, they allowed me to present one slide in advance to check that the content was audible and clear. This advance check made me feel so much more at ease.

TOP TIP

✓ Walk yourself through the process and have a think about everything you may need while reflecting on any previous interview and assessment experiences. Do you need extra time? Do you need the questions before you arrive?

If you know the interview questions in advance, this can help with a multitude of access requirements, fatigue, anxiety, pain, AAC needs, and even sensory needs, for starters. This is one of the simplest ways to meet access needs, yet it's such a rarity. Having the questions in advance in a profession like occupational therapy doesn't give disabled applicants an advantage over non-disabled applicants as this knowledge should be based on getting to know you as an occupational therapist, and shouldn't be Googleable! In fact, it shouldn't matter, disability or not – we should all have this access. We encourage students to develop reflective practice skills at university as an integral part of their personal and professional development, yet we're pressuring them to think on the spot during an interview. I know sometimes you may need quick thinking, but this doesn't really add up, does it?

I always go to an interview with an idea of how many hours I would want to work, knowing that my fatigue levels cannot handle a full-time job. For others, full-time employment may work, and this may be something they enjoy or they may not have another option. You could make this work with flexible working hours and days. During my first role at the University of Huddersfield I did four days, during which I travelled onsite for three days and my fourth day was used to work remotely, online. This really helped my energy and pain levels. Flexible working enabled me to be the occupational therapist I wanted to be. Also, the remote working hours were perfect to either put in additional hours or finish early depending on how my work schedule had panned out that week. This certainly helped when it came to Friday afternoons if I'd done a longer day throughout the week!

If you are like me and not only prefer but need part-time work to manage your health, then this can be hard to find. *News flash!* Not every Band 5 occupational therapist is a young, non-disabled person, or any band or grade for that matter! This totally frustrated me when job hunting because every role I found would be full-time, and those that said full-time or part-time working were never actually that open to part-time working when I emailed them to enquire. I used to ask about hours in my email prior to the interview, although now I wouldn't. I say impress them first, and then talk about this when they ask you about your working preferences after the interview. As someone who's always had a plan and felt the need to disclose, this was a hard one, but if the recruitment team really want you, they will put that flexible working/job share into place as again, this should classify as a reasonable adjustment.

I do understand, though, that this is not as straightforward as it sounds, and if you're new to the world of work it can be hard establishing the pattern that works for you and your energy levels. Personally I work better in the morning, and find that my energy levels take quite the dip during the afternoon, whereas others may work better in the afternoon. Have these open and honest discussions with your potential employer if the role allows flexibility, as you never know what may be able to be adapted to suit you (sorry to sound like a broken record).

So let's imagine you have the job (congratulations!). The next step is going to occupational health. After my rather ableist experience of occupational health getting into university, the thought of going through this again when I got my first postgraduate job made me feel sick to the stomach. Even worse was that this one was to be done over the phone. I mean, at least I didn't have to waste my energy travelling, but at the back of my mind I thought that this wasn't going to go down well given my speech impairment. To my surprise, though, it was the best occupational health experience!

I'd explained to my manager a month prior, before this assessment was due, how nervous I was to go through the process of getting the job. The manager suggested that I put down as much detail as I thought I needed on the form before I had my appointment with occupational health. I decided to take the approach of writing down the adjustments I needed on my previous placement, and essentially copied my pre-place-ment learning agreement I had had at university (see the example in Chapter Six), and it worked like a charm.

When the phone call appointment took place I picked up the phone to the loveliest assessor, who was certainly in the right job. I was not only listened to, but I was understood – literally, medically and personally. The assessor recognized that I knew my needs best, as this process of writing my needs down enabled me to show them that I knew what I was talking about, and I appreciated that. Let's be honest – if you're an occupational therapist with a long-term health condition yourself, then you know your stuff. However, the assessor knew that I didn't have all the answers for every single day of work, as chronic pain and fatigue fluctuates; it was so refreshing to have someone understand the variation of needs that come with chronic illness! However, I think that this should be the norm rather than refreshing, and you shouldn't have to give someone all your medical history for this to happen.

I personally disclosed quite a bit before that appointment, such as fatigue, and even things like the fact that using a pair of scissors was hard for me. But medically I didn't go into much detail other than disclosing my cerebral palsy. I was very careful not to go into too much unnecessary detail on the principle that I don't owe anyone my medical history. Everyone varies as to how much personal medical information they prefer to give out and for some, what I disclose may seem a lot to disclose medically. It also does seem like a negative introduction to showcase your struggles, illustrating what you can or can't do. I actually offer so much more because of my experience of disability, which needs to be acknowledged (again, refer to Chapter Six). On reflection I probably disclosed too much despite being careful, but I'd rather do it this way than experience the same as my occupational health appointment at university!

I certainly did not need to inform occupational health that I drive an adapted vehicle, but at this point Dad was still sat at the side of me while I drove to Huddersfield and back to Sheffield (and probably still is as you read this), so it was important, and the most worrying part of me starting work, as I wasn't even considering jobs out of Sheffield to begin with. But disclosing my adapted vehicle was beneficial as it allowed me to discuss my parking needs. This also enabled me to go through Access to Work to get help with getting to and from work and transferring my wheelchair in and out of the car (GOV.UK n.d.).

Scope (2023) has an insightful page that tells you everything you need to know about the minefield of **Access to Work**.

Since starting work, I have become so much more confident at driving, and have even started to enjoy my commute to work (with Dad). I think it just took me more practice and time than some new drivers; perhaps due to my hand controls and disability, and perhaps due to the fact that I am a perfectionist who loves to do each task really well. I now feel that I can confidently say that I am a good driver, and am much better at adapting this experience, such as focusing on navigation and physical motor control even when I am fatigued. Dad is around more for getting to work than I envisioned he would be, I will admit, due to circumstances, but I've accepted this, and am very lucky that as a family we can manage this.

As you can see there's a lot more that goes into finding a job when you have a disability, and mine was quite the journey, so much so that I am not looking forward to the day that I move on from the University of Huddersfield as I know there'll be more red tape. But just remember that you know your needs best because there's no other greater advocate than yourself. I most definitely leaned on to help me through this time, which badly impacted my mental health. But I am glad that I stuck with it and found a job that allows me to fly – not only as an occupational therapist, but also as a disabled activist.

I hope that this chapter has helped you to navigate this complex time, if this has happened to you. If this did happen, what did you do? What suggestions can you make to change this process?

As for employers, have you ever interviewed anyone with a disability? How is your recruitment process? How would you have handled this situation in your organization? What systems and processes need to be changed?

NOT SO TERRIBLE...P.A.L.S.Y. REFLECTIVE LOG
Pausing
Stop and think about what you have read in this chapter. What are your main takeaway points? What are your main questions?

. . . .

. . . .

. . . .

Analysing
Why did this resonate with you?

. . . .

. . . .

. . . .

Learning
What did you learn from this?

....

....

....

Solving
What actions need to be put into place?

....

....

....

Your plan
How will you achieve these actions? What are your goals?

....

....

....

References

Duncan, E.A.S. (2021) *Foundations for Practice in Occupational Therapy* (6th edn). Edinburgh: Elsevier.

DWP (Department for Work and Pensions) (2021) *Disability Confident Employer Scheme.* Collection. London: DWP. Accessed on 27 December 2022 at www.gov.uk/government/collections/disability-confident-campaign

GOV.UK (no date) *Access to Work: Get Support If You Have a Disability or Health Condition.* Accessed on 27 December 2022 at www.gov.uk/access-to-work

Kumari Campbell, F. (2009) 'Internalised Ableism: The Tyranny Within.' In F. Kumari Campbell, *Contours of Ableism: The Production of Disability and Abledness* (pp.16–29). London: Palgrave Macmillan.

Marks, D. (1999) *Disability: Controversial Debates and Psychosocial Perspectives.* London: Routledge.

NHS (National Health Service) (2019) 'Chapter 2: More NHS action on prevention and health inequalities.' In *Online Version of the NHS Long Term Plan.* Accessed on 20 December 2022 at www.longtermplan.nhs.uk/online-version/chapter-2-more-nhs-action-on-prevention-and-health-inequalities

Scope (2023) 'Access to Work grant scheme.' Accessed on 19 April 2023 at www.scope.org.uk/advice-and-support/access-to-work-grant-scheme/

CHAPTER ELEVEN

Re-Evaluating Activism as an Occupation

Despite how great it is to see people read and reflect on my ableist experiences, I always come back to the same question... Does this blog have enough impact to create change?

I remember having huge imposter syndrome when I was asked to write this book and, truth be told, I still have this. But I think that the opportunity has been great to cement and re-evaluate my activism.

I am so glad that I started my blog – it has been such a powerful tool for my own learning. Since I started it as a more light-hearted lifestyle blog, I still have a varied audience. Some readers come to find out about my experiences as a disabled occupational therapist, but others are more interested in my life in general. Perhaps this is because they can relate to me, are parents to a child with cerebral palsy, or they're just quite fond of me (let's face it, I am awesome). Joking aside, though, my blog now appeals to a wide audience. Since my initial intention was just to raise awareness of cerebral palsy, I still can't quite believe this. I owe it to my amazing readers to produce varied content, and creating such a variety is so much fun.

I love producing more conversational content, but when unpicking complicated reflections, I often find it difficult to be snappy and concise. This then often limits the depth of my analysis and reflections due to word count constraints and modifying content to suit a range of audiences.

During my time waiting to become a registered occupational therapist and finding a job, I analysed my life experiences a lot, and I truly believe that this period of retrospection enabled me to move forward in my career. Although these six months were tough, having the opportunity to speak at events after qualifying motivated me to make my activism more robust. Since this period, my activism has shifted enormously and I find myself questioning my own practice and activism more. Don't get me wrong, though – I love writing for my blog *Not So Terrible Palsy*,[1] and this will always be my go-to for rambles and personal stories.

Despite how great it is to see people read and reflect on my ableist experiences, I always come back to the same question... Does this blog have enough impact to create change?

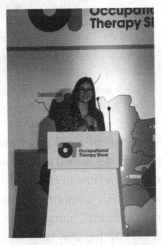

Image 11.1. *Georgia, a white woman, standing on stage at a conference in a black dress with a white pattern, wearing glasses. The stand in front of her reads 'Occupational Therapy Show'.*

I genuinely do believe that if I went straight into work on qualifying, I wouldn't be here. Yes, I may still be writing a book, having been approached to put this book proposal together shortly after finishing my degree, but I would have just written a book full of my experiences. While this would still be valid, that crucial critical layer would be missing. I'm going round in circles here, as these life experiences are, in fact, necessary in order to provide this platform. Analysing my activism this way can be difficult at times and poses a lot of questions. How did I get here? Why do others need to hear about my life experiences? Writing

---

1   https://notsoterriblepalsy.com

with all of these questions in mind has been one of the most useful outlets so far to help me address where my activism started and, most importantly, to re-evaluate where it's going.

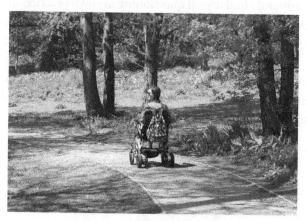

Image 11.2. *Georgia, a white female, wheeling off along a path surrounded by greenery. She is seated in a black, powered wheelchair.*

For example, in the first part of this book I used my experiences as an occupational therapist and disabled activist to critically explore my childhood experiences and my time in children's services. Yes, I utilized my own lived experiences, but would I even be aware of the pitfalls in practice without my disability? Alongside my disabled experience, being involved in AbleOTUK[2] has also helped enhance my knowledge massively. AbleOTUK is part of a bigger affinity network alongside LGBTQIA+OTUK[3] and BAMEOTUK (for Black, Asian and Minoritized Ethnicities).[4] All three affinity groups work together closely alongside the Royal College of Occupational Therapists (RCOT) to challenge the profession through an intersectional lens, teaching me so much about forms of diversity within my profession. But would I have come to any of the conclusions that I've drawn in this book solely from using knowledge from my degree without factoring in my disability? No.

This is because the occupational therapy profession doesn't give you the tools to challenge practice. In fact, it gives very little indication that practice needs disrupting in the first place. I am not just saying this as a

2   https://affinot.co.uk/ableotuk
3   https://affinot.co.uk/lgbtqiaotuk
4   www.bameot.uk

criticism as I know more discourse is happening surrounding disrupting practice, and that this is a current cultural shift in the profession. This profession is so diverse that training could not possibly prepare you for every area of practice, never mind how to question that practice, and as for practice, I know the job is demanding, but if you're reading this book, you know changes need to be made.

How can we learn to make changes by being allies and disruptors in the profession when we are not given the correct tools to do so in practice or in education? I can recall as many stories as I like about my experiences, but if I don't indicate how change can happen and give others something tangible to work with, how does that actually challenge ableism? We need to work as a collective to create spaces in occupational therapy practice for allyship. This will then create the tools to overcome the pragmatic challenges of ableist systems and discrimination, enabling qualified professionals and students to confidently call out discrimination.

Before we create change, we must understand allyship. This is a key concept that we've addressed throughout this book. There are multiple protected characteristics under the Equality Act 2010, which include: age, disability, race, gender reassignment, marriage and civil partnership, pregnancy and maternity, religion or belief, sex and sexual orientation (Equality and Human Rights Commission 2021), so remember, we all have protected characteristics, it's just that some have more than others. Therefore, we must consider intersectionality and other health inequalities. As a cisgendered, white woman I have privileges and I can only speak from my limited experiences when covering the concepts of diversity and belonging, but I can still be an ally to those with other protected characteristics from this position of privilege.

Nicole Asong Nfonoyim-Hara, Director of the Diversity Programs at Mayo Clinic, defines allyship as 'when a person of privilege works in solidarity and partnership with a marginalized group of people to help take down the systems that challenge that group's basic rights, equal access, and ability to thrive in our society' (Nfonoyim-Hara, cited in Dickenson 2021). Samantha-Rae Dickenson, Diversity, Equity, and Inclusion Director for Goodwill Industries International, Inc., takes this further by adding that allies must also have a degree of power in order to spark change (2021).

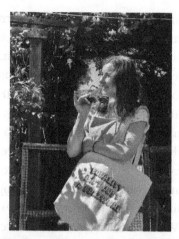

Image 11.3. *Georgia, a white female, stood outdoors surrounded by greenery. She is looking to the right holding her sunglasses and is wearing dungaree shorts. She has a bag on her left shoulder that is designed by the charity Scope, which reads 'EQUALITY ISN'T JUST A BUZZWORD'.*

Being an ally is so important and is a key recurring theme in talks at national conferences from BAMEOTUK, AbleOTUK and LGBTQIA+OT UK. To be an ally, you need to learn, listen and advocate (Inclusive Employers n.d.). It's key to learn from us, but also to do your own research too. I'm not saying that you have to drown yourself in research; I understand that everyone has other priorities and a life to manage. Whatever the reason you're reading this, learning is lifelong and the initial research is readily available. I still have a lot of learning to do about ableism through my own research, never mind other forms of discrimination that I don't personally experience. Listen to us and believe us; many people don't believe our stories and choose not to comprehend them since our life experiences aren't relatable to them. Well, this world isn't perfect and negative experiences do happen.

Listen to our stories because some are pretty hard to tell, and believe us as this then means we can form collective activism through allyship. We're all stronger together, right? Allyship is a meaningful occupation (Pywell *et al.* 2022), which requires you to advocate and act. I'm not asking you to shout from the rooftops if that's not your thing (unlike me) – advocacy can be as small or as big as you'd like and still make an impact. Examples of advocacy are: reflecting on your behaviours, calling out inappropriate behaviours or discrimination, sharing opportunities and listening to feedback from those with lived experience (Inclusive Employers n.d.).

I can be an ally to you through sharing my research. Read 'What is allyship? A quick guide' (Inclusive Employers n.d.) to enhance your own activism.

Let's use language and terminology as an example of how you can be an ally; yes, it's time to have the 'people with disabilities' vs. 'disabled people' debate. I personally prefer to be referred to as a 'disabled person'. This is because the term 'people *with* disabilities' places the responsibility on the individual to attain higher levels of function themselves through managing their own health (Whalley Hammell 2022). The concept of becoming 'less disabled' is then the focus, rather than addressing the limitations that attitudinal barriers, physical environments and structures are placing on disabled people (Whalley Hammell 2022). Now I'm aware that how people want to be addressed is a personal choice and neither term can be called ableist; this is why I've used both phrases throughout this book. Just because you have experience of disability doesn't mean you're automatically a perfect ally to disabled people!

Asking for people's preferred terminology is something simple that can be done in practice, just like you would ask someone for their pronouns. Without enforcing this, it could even be an option box to fill out during the initial assessment stage within the occupational therapy process. For example:

Is one of these terms relevant to your lived experiences?

☐ A disabled person

☐ A person with a disability

☐ A person with lived experience

☐ A person with a long-term or chronic health condition

☐ None of the above

☐ Other (please specify) _____

How each person labels themselves is a very personal choice; we may choose to be labelled as a 'disabled person', a 'person with disabilities' or even not to use the title 'disabled' at all. There is also the potential that occupational therapists may not even know the importance of using the correct language and terminology. As a profession that works with many disabled people, we can't ignore the importance of language and terminology, and we must act as allies and do the learning. Yes, you might not get this right the first time, but allyship is a learning process, and showing willingness to learn from your mistakes is key – no one is perfect.

I certainly don't know if what I've suggested throughout this book will make a difference; we all get it wrong at times, and this is why using research enables me to make more credible links and improve my own understanding of what is quite a complicated social, environmental and political situation. I'm a woman in my early twenties and am by no means an expert in this. I don't have a degree in disability studies and nine times out of ten I don't get paid to do the freelance work I do. Sometimes I don't even know if I'm doing the right thing – I can't tell you how many times I've re-written paragraphs in this book.

How do I address this huge systemic problem and move the issues forward? An occupation is something that a person wants to or needs to *do* in order to live or enhance their life. Rights refer to 'doing more than having' (Young 1990, p.25), which places occupational therapists in a unique position to address occupational rights and challenge the concepts of moral relativism, thus enhancing wellbeing (Whalley Hammell and Iwama 2011), such as providing a service user with a mobility aid to enable their right to movement and easier access to society. The fulfilment of these occupational rights, which all individuals need to engage in for survival, such as eating, is called 'occupational justice' (WFOT 2019). Occupational injustice is when these needs are not being met, but this concept doesn't address why these occupations are being unfulfilled and the inequality behind this (Hammell and Iwama 2012). Therefore, we cannot create change without addressing these causes of inequality and considering the history.

I went into my studies without knowing the history of the profession and the systemic flaws, and not really having a political mindset. I was simply a 19-year-old living my life day-by-day. I started my blog about being a disabled occupational therapy student, not realizing that the concepts I was blogging about had so much systemic history. All right, I knew that I wasn't alone in feeling oppressed by the system, but I didn't realize how deeply broken the system actually was. It is well known that historically the profession has been, and still is, dominated by white, middle-class, heterosexual, cisgendered, non-disabled females. We must acknowledge this history and change the record. If we don't acknowledge this, how do we avoid history repeating itself? For example, I didn't fully acknowledge these systemic flaws until I gained my role as a graduate teaching assistant at the University of Huddersfield. Supporting in lectures gave me a perspective of academia beyond being a student learner, as I could now clearly see the institutional barriers within practice.

I know that I am a slow learner, and it is only my passion towards addressing ableism in the profession that makes this minefield easier for me to grasp. This poses the question as to whether I needed to see and even experience some of these systemic injustices for myself to make sense of them. Furthermore, were these concepts perhaps not explicitly analysed during my studies? I'm not saying that we all have to be experts in occupational justice, but if I, as a disabled person and qualified occupational therapist, am only just managing to relate context to theory, then how conflicting must it feel for those who are unaware that they are experiencing ableism?

Addressing the systemic issues within the occupational therapy profession makes the whole world a better place. Makes your head hurt, right? I know. But if we are all occupational beings, like Wilcox (1993) suggests, then this is why disrupting ableism in the occupational therapy profession is so vital – not just for the profession itself, but also for wider society, whether they know about occupational science and its influences or not.

So how far have we come as a profession in recognizing this standpoint? **Sam Pywell**, a qualified occupational therapist working in academia, explores this:

Ableism exists in the OT [occupational therapy] profession. Once you see it, you understand it's a threshold concept and that you've crossed into this other dimension that not everyone sees. Equally, you can't go back as it changes your viewpoint. You then listen to colleagues and students talking who don't understand or see ableism and think, my goodness...in my profession...out of all professions...no. Then the shame hits you like a brick wall. I was ashamed of what I heard. I felt ashamed to be an OT [occupational therapist] at one point. Then I moved forward...it took time, reflection and learning about anti-ableist practices... and now I'm acting and active in that space of addressing it.

Yep, I've naively thought this too – surely if those I'm working with have more understanding of disability then I will be working in a much more supportive environment? That's not always the case. I'm not saying I've been totally unsupported as the environment that I am currently working in is super-supportive. But there are a lot of disabled occupational therapists out there who are facing a lot of ableism daily. We know this now, we've heard the stories, and we can no longer hide behind *'but I'm an occupational therapist, I cannot be ableist'*. I'm not explicitly calling any specific occupational therapist ableist; I'm just here to call out ableist practices. Qualifying within this profession doesn't automatically make you anti-ableist, and you should still always make sure you're questioning your practice. We've all probably been ableist at some point in our lives; it's now time to recognize this and to do something about it.

So what intervention is needed? The intervention within this book is the reflective log included at the end of each chapter. This shows how seamless it can be to analyse your own learning processes. It focuses on reflecting on *your* learning and how this applies to *you* in the hope that *you* can contextualize these complicated systemic issues. Once these issues are contextualized, which is not easy and takes time, then *you* can create *tangible* action points to do something about it. Highlighting your learning does not mean I am calling you ableist; we all have learning to do and need to be reflecting to keep up with the changes in practice. Addressing ableism and other systemic inequities is everyone's business, and we need to be doing this as individuals and as an occupational therapy profession globally.

DisruptOT[5] is an international community that moves beyond this reflection and actively challenges this status quo of institutional discrimination within the occupational therapy profession.

---

5   www.disruptot.org

Find out how you can get involved to drive this change within practice.

DisruptOT influenced me greatly. I felt very privileged to be asked to do a week-long takeover of the DisruptOT Twitter account in 2022. This actually started off Occupational Therapy Month with them in April, which was epic. But in the weeks prior to the takeover, I was so nervous. Yes, I had a few stories to share and I knew how to generate discussions, but it made me reflect on whether my activism was enough. At the time I had just submitted the proposal for this book so I was experiencing huge imposter syndrome anyway, and re-evaluating if my activism was having the right impact. I'm so lucky that my passion had played a huge role in the direction of my career. As I have had the opportunity to speak about ableism on some great platforms, those I have spoken to may have been impacted by my work, and I hope that my work has resonated with them to make changes within their own practice. But how do I know this for sure? How can I even be sure that this book will do anything to help reduce the amount of ableism faced in practice? This uncertainty makes it so easy to give up – I can't tell you how many times I've thought about giving up on this very book. The truth is, I can only be confident in my work and activism if I have allies. I will never address all ableism in this book, because dismantling ableism is beyond my control, and interventions must be carried out and evaluated by collective action.

Collective action – we have landed here yet again. The concept of a collective perspective goes back to the idea of interdependence (Malfitano, Whiteford and Molineux 2019). Since we are all interconnected, a small change within practice can have more widespread repercussions than we initially might think. For example, within children's services, an occupational therapist can have a widespread effect on not only the child but also the school and how they adapt their thinking processes or physical buildings or social environments to suit other students' needs. We need to be constantly thinking about our effect in the present and how this will have repercussions in the future.

Collectivism and individualism have influenced the development of occupational therapy in so many ways (Malfitano *et al.* 2019). I can see why both of these perspectives are so crucial to have because we are all individuals, yet we are influenced by and shaped from collective experiences. Both collectivism and individualism are important within person-centred practice – everyone has the right to choose occupations that are meaningful to them, their community and overarching social perspective. But occupational therapists deliver services and, although the aim is to engage individuals in meaningful occupations, systemic injustices continue to exist and must be looked at collectively to evaluate framework and policy (Malfitano *et al.* 2019).

I have tried to suggest an action that can be done for most points I've made during this book, for instance the signposting given above to DisruptOT, to help you in your disruption and research journey, and the example of the question surrounding how a person with lived experienced wants to be referred to – these are two very tangible action points you can follow within your own practice, right? But some of the other ideologies I've spoken about are a lot harder to address, such as my personal experiences of getting an EHCP. Yes, I've made a few suggestions along the way, and my parents' story has hopefully made it clearer on what needs to change and why, but my working-class parents and myself alone aren't going to change the system, frameworks and policies. We need collective activism, so the relationship between macro structures, policies, politics, rights and citizenship must be central to occupational therapy practice (Malfitano *et al.* 2019). For example, I can only advocate from my perspective within occupational therapy, so I require a multidisciplinary team to reinforce my work with service users, enabling the picture to be addressed holistically.

We've established that we need to work together and that as a profession we have the correct tools to do this because occupational therapists are awesome and can change the world! But we don't have all the answers, and if this change is to progress correctly through collectivism and allyship, we must work with others. So who are you going to work with and what is your main priority? Can you turn your learning and priorities into tangible actions? What are you going to include in your action plan within the 'Not So Terrible...P.A.L.S.Y.' reflective log?

If you want to share your tangible action points, please do. Use the hashtag #ChallengingAbleismInHealthcare. We can all be allies and learn from one another and, most importantly act on this!

NOT SO TERRIBLE...P.A.L.S.Y. REFLECTIVE LOG
Pausing
Stop and think about what you have read in this chapter. What are your main takeaway points? What are your main questions?

. . . .

. . . .

. . . .

Analysing
Why did this resonate with you?

. . . .

. . . .

. . . .

Learning
What did you learn from this?

. . . .

. . . .

. . . .

Solving
What actions need to be put into place?

. . . .

. . . .

. . . .

Your plan
How will you achieve these actions? What are your goals?

. . . .

. . . .

. . . .

References

Dickenson, S.-R. (2021) 'What is allyship?' *Communities*, 28 January. Accessed on 29 December 2022 at www.edi.nih.gov/blog/communities/what-allyship

DisruptOT (2022) 'DisruptOT: How it started and how it's going!' [Video] May. Accessed on 16 February 2023 at www.youtube.com/watch?v=AWcwF4FfbOl

Equality and Human Rights Commission (2021) 'Protected characteristics.' Accessed on 11 February 2023 at www.equalityhumanrights.com/en/equality-act/protected-characteristics

Inclusive Employers (no date) 'What is allyship? A quick guide.' *Inclusion Allies* [Blog]. Accessed on 30 December 2022 at www.inclusiveemployers.co.uk/blog/quick-guide-to-allyship

Malfitano, A. P. S., Whiteford, G. and Molineux, M. (2019). 'Transcending the individual: The promise and potential of collectivist approaches in occupational therapy.' *Scandinavian Journal of Occupational Therapy 28*, 3, 188–200. Accessed on17 February 2023 at https://doi.org/10.1080/11038128.2019.1693627

Pywell, S., Hicks, N., Vine, G. and Booth-Gardiner, R. (2022) 'Allyship – It's Time to Make It a Meaningful Occupation!' Occupational Therapy Show, 24 November, Birmingham.

WFOT (World Federation of Occupational Therapists) (2019) Position Statement on Human Rights. Accessed on 24 July 2023 at https://wfot.org/resources/occupational-therapy-and-human-rights

Whalley Hammell, K. (2022) 'A call to resist occupational therapy's promotion of ableism.' *Scandinavian Journal of Occupational Therapy.* Accessed on 1 January 2023 at https://doi.org/10.1080/11038128.2022.2130821

Whalley Hammell, K. and Iwama, M.K. (2011) 'Well-being and occupational rights: An imperative for critical occupational therapy.' *Scandinavian Journal of Occupational Therapy 19*, 5, 385–394. Accessed on 17 February 2023 at www.tandfonline.com/doi/abs/10.3109/11038128.2011.611821?journalCode=iocc20

Wilcox, A. (1993) 'A theory of the human need for occupation.' *Journal of Occupational Science 1*, 1, 17–24. Accessed on 14 January 2023 at https://doi.org/10.1080/14427591.1993.9686375

Young, I.M. (1990) *Justice and the Politics of Difference.* Princeton, NJ: Princeton University Press.

CHAPTER TWELVE

Thinking Critically About My Future as a Disabled Occupational Therapist

Even negative experiences or ableism have become pinnacle learning opportunities that I can now utilize in my disabled activism and also feed back to those starting their occupational therapy training.

Considering lived experience is vital to analyse societal and systemic discrimination, yet my singular perspective has only allowed me to cover certain aspects of disability, so it's important to refer to others with their own lived experiences. No two experiences of disability are the same, which is why I considered a range of perspectives, including children's occupational therapists, those with lived experience of cerebral palsy, students, academics and newly qualified occupational therapists. So have you got your critical lens ready? Can any of these points be transferrable to your area of practice or life experience?

Occupational therapy within children's services

Going back to the start, then, what are the main points to address ableism within children's services?

Deborah Bergel, through her lived experience of disability, explores this:

> The two occupational therapists who worked with me as a child were sweet and patient women who made sure occupational therapy was fun; I remember feeling like they provided a safe space. I have always

struggled with dexterity and pain, even after I learned to hold a pencil comfortably. Yet my occupational therapist was still focused on making my handwriting more legible, trying to make me hold pencils like the 'norm'. This led to great frustration for both me and my parents. The excessive focus on writing led my therapists to neglect other skills such as hair care and finding accessible alternatives. This is more important to me now and caused difficulties once I left home and couldn't use a comb without being in pain or tangling my hair.

As I grew up, I became interested in music even though my left hand made playing instruments difficult. Yet the cultures I grew up in tend to stigmatize disability and don't centre accessibility, so I was never given adaptive opportunities to learn music by my schools or my therapists. It is only through receiving adaptive music lessons at college and playing the piano that my fine motor skills have improved. I wish my occupational therapists had focused on things other than making me write in a way that was considered 'normal'. Adaptive pencil grips to enable me to hold my pencil 'correctly' benefited me and shouldn't have been questioned. I wish I had been supported earlier to build up other skills that were meaningful to me.

Reading this really struck a chord with me because it's clear that what is being talked about here are bottom-up approaches. Reflecting on my experiences in children's services, I was aware of the less meaningful and impactful interventions that I received. Due to my occupational therapy training, I can now contextualize these flaws further. It's clear to me that disabled people are unknowingly aware of the flaws of the bottom-up approach, so we need to be questioning our practice. We must be continuously analysing our standpoint, including during the intervention stage of the occupational therapy process, asking questions such as: am I using a top-down approach? Am I thinking about occupations that are meaningful to the person rather than using the 'hierarchy of occupations' (Yao et al. 2022, p.7)?

Progress is constant, and Deborah's international perspective might vary from those within the UK. There is even a wide variety of experience within the UK with a 'postcode lottery' when it comes to getting support like EHCPs, never mind the global differences. Yet cultural norms and expectations are still forcing people into boxes. I, too, play the piano, and I only started this with lots of encouragement since my internalized ableism gave me the perspective that *I couldn't do that* in the 'normal way'. There's no singular way to play the piano. Therefore, we not only have to challenge these issues systemically; we also have to challenge our beliefs so that disabled children know that anything is possible, even if they are achieved in a different way. We're a beautiful, diverse population, and we need to embrace that in order for everyone to achieve their dreams. Yes, it sounds cheesy, and yes, there are other political issues to tackle, but attitudes are a big part of what we need to address. This is why we must challenge perceptions and increase representation. Representation has such a profound effect, and we must never stop striving towards accurate representation so that those in the disabled community are never made to feel limited. For me, chronic pain and fatigue do get in the way, but I'm in control of these limits, just like we are all in control of changing our attitudes.

Faith Newton, occupational therapist and author of *Inclusive PE for SEND Children* (2023), addresses this:

> As OTs [occupational therapists] we need to be confident enough to work with school leadership to change systems. Instead of working with individual children to 'fix' their deficits, we need to be changing policies, environments and teaching methods to be more inclusive. Practically, this means learning the language and world view of education, understanding Ofsted requirements and letting school leadership know what we can offer. We have so much to bring to the whole school approach and yet we get stuck doing puzzles.

Representation and improving attitudes is one thing, but changing systems is another. I am in a privileged position, I'm not going to deny that, and I don't know what effect this book will have yet. However, if policies and systems don't change, it becomes very hard for a shift to happen. These conversations only come up when something is publicized or happens to the disabled community; we all get on our soapbox to discuss something for a short period until it's then compartmentalized, and that particular topic gets put on the top shelf, as do our soapboxes. But for the disabled community, our soapboxes can never truly be put away because this is our reality. We need allies to be on this continuous journey with us, and stop putting conversations on the back-burner because the more waves we make, the greater the likelihood of policy makers and leaders listening. We need you – please don't pick and choose your solidarity because that isn't actually solidarity. To reach those who can make that change, we must keep waving that flag, continually questioning ableist practice. In the quote above, Faith is right – Ofsted should utilize all the tools that occupational therapists have in order to create a more inclusive educational system.

Lee Ridley, more commonly known as the Lost Voice Guy, speaks about this:

> I would like to see more support given to people after they leave educa-
> tion. I was pretty well supported until I left my SEN [special educational
> needs] school but afterwards I felt that I dropped off the radar a bit. It's
> only more recently that I've found out about services and other stuff
> that may be of assistance to me, but I found all of this out by myself.

Laura Casey, who has a lived experience of cerebral palsy, expands on this, saying:

> CP [cerebral palsy] is a lifelong condition; however, according to the
> healthcare system, it appears to disappear once you turn 18! The service
> pathways stop! As a service user (and an OT!) this is incredibly frus-
> trating as, with no adult pathway for CP, you need to shout loud for
> support you require. Not receiving the right ongoing support has had
> a big impact on my function as an adult, even though technically CP is
> not a progressive condition. This has caused a lot of stress and isolation
> at times, so needs to change.

Of course, the transition into adulthood was going to come up when I asked people with cerebral palsy how practice can be improved – there are reasons for my rambles! I know how it feels to leave children's ser-vices, and it's not a period of my life that I'd like to re-live; you certainly do feel 'dropped', as Lee calls it. Yet actually, this feeling and stress don't ever go away because every hurdle reminds you that you're navigating life without the support of an EHCP. As Laura points out, our needs and access requirements change over time. Mine have, and dealing with these changes is hard. Every adult's life has its challenges, but it can be so mentally and physically exhausting having to research services and navigate through red tape. I agree with Laura when she says you feel like you have to shout the loudest just to receive support to enable you to live the life that you want.

This is another reason why finding the disabled community and connecting with people with lived experience of cerebral palsy was so important to me because it validated my experience. I realized that these experiences weren't just me being 'picky' or 'ungrateful'; they were systemic flaws that most disabled people experience. We aren't being ungrateful; we just know our rights, and we deserve to live a fulfilling life. I know the correct intentions are there and, in an ideal world, systems would be different, but it's time to stop hiding behind the future 'ideal world' because change needs to happen now. I know systemic changes can't happen overnight, but it's time to get the ball rolling and persist regardless of whether these are 'hot topics' or not.

Occupational therapy studies

Natalie Hicks, an occupational therapist in-training, explores anti-ableist practice:

> OTs should not be judgemental. If a student or another OT is struggling, consider, prior to assuming the worst, that they may be neurodivergent, struggling with their mental health or have an invisible illness. You can ask them if they are okay and whether they need support. It is best to be a kind person and help rather than judging someone without knowing the facts.

You never know who may have a hidden disability and yes, while I've discussed positive disclosure, it is still up to that individual to choose whether to disclose or not. We need to think before we make assumptions about students. Imagine having just been given a diagnosis of a health condition and having no idea how to address this. Some of us can't, and we will never know until we're in that position. I certainly don't have all the answers either. It is about being a kind and approachable person in order to help that student with whatever it is that they're going through. You see, it's not that hard to act as an ally.

Jeantique Hommel, a disabled occupational therapy student, discusses this further:

Disclosing my disabilities and autism at university has made my experience so much harder because of the discrimination and obstacles it has led to. A few things that would have helped me so much at university include:

- Embedding disability awareness training into the curriculum, for example inviting disabled guest lecturers to talk about their experiences as AHPs (allied healthcare professionals) and/or service users. Another helpful option would be to provide reflective opportunities for peers to think about how they can support students with different access needs throughout the duration of the course.

- Having the option to meet my personal tutor more often to discuss issues specific to my access needs (without this time eating into academic tutorials).

- Being provided with a 'disability passport' system so that all lecturers could be aware of my individual access needs so that I didn't have to create and send one myself.

- Having a 'disability representative' from my course who can work alongside cohort representatives (but in a more accessible and self-defined role) to feed back about specific accessibility-related issues.

- Trusting that I know my access needs best and adapting to my suggestions, not ignoring them in favour of lecturers' own preferences.

Overall, fostering a culture where disabilities and differences are not just accepted but also actually celebrated would make so much of a difference! I know that my disabilities will make me a better OT, but I'm still working on having to 'prove' to everyone around me at university that this is genuinely true!

So many tangible action points here! If you struggled writing your reflection at the end of the last chapter, then hopefully this will give you some inspiration. The point that stood out to me the most was inclusion of disabled guest lecturers within the course programme – genuinely, guest lecturing is one of my favourite parts about the work that I do as it's so rewarding!

Griffiths (2020, 2020a) hosted an #OTalk on Twitter and found that 33 per cent of occupational therapists have never heard of ableism. I remember participating in this #OTalk and being stunned by the results of the polls. Since then, AbleOTUK has been formed and is generating these conversations on its platforms regularly, so I should hope that these figures have changed. AbleOTUK provides important resources and networks to whom I can direct enquiries after my guest lecturing, in order for students to further their allyship and learning. I find guest lecturing enriching as it allows me to see students begin to contextualize ableism and then understand where ableism could arise in everyday practice. Implementing this critical perspective in training is so crucial. Whenever I'm supporting in a seminar, I always add my perspective. I'm aware that it's my opinion and I would never force my views on others, but I've found it really helps students to begin to look at practice through an anti-discriminatory lens. Students now know when I'm going to chip in and give my perspective as a disabled person as they are becoming more aware of these concepts. I can be on my soapbox all day, but if those I'm preaching to aren't even aware how to recognize ableist practices, then nothing is going to get done about it, is it?

Now I can't speak for every university as I know some universities already have specific tutors who are the disability leads, but I guess it's about asking ourselves what more can be done. Some of the suggestions I've made in this book you may already be doing, or you may have something different put into place that works better for your learning environment. We need to constantly be analysing these systems. Are they doing what they set out to do? Are there any recurring problems? Is there anything else that can be implemented? If you're an academic, why don't you ask students these questions yourself and, if you're a student, is there anything you'd like to take forward to your course lead? You know your access needs better than anyone else!

Occupational therapy practice

Devyn Awalt, an occupational therapist with cerebral palsy, discusses what an anti-ableist practice might look like:

Anti-ableist practice to me is giving me the opportunity to prove that I can do the job...as a person with CP, I can provide a unique lived experience with the people we help. We can be and are great OTs.

Jay Webster, an occupational therapist, furthers this discussion:

Anti-ableist practice to me is creating space for people to be their authentic selves and to have what they need in place to enable them to be the best occupational therapist that they can be, no questions asked. If someone says they need an accommodation, then give it to them and ensure they are supported so that they can support others in their work.

Simplistically, this is all I want and all anyone desires, right, just to be appreciated? I am appreciated in the current role that I am in now and I am valued, not just because I can use my lived experience to aid my practice, but because I'm good at my job. These two quotes really bring it home for me. Yes, I want my lived experience to be valued because it's what makes me the occupational therapist I am. I'm not good at my job *in despite of* my cerebral palsy; I'm good at my job *with* my cerebral palsy. With the correct space and tools, you will see me thrive! As disabled people, we just want to be valued.

Robyn, an occupational therapist with a disability, highlights inclusion in the workplace:

It is ironic that, as occupational therapists we are about problem-solving and yet my experience of working as an occupational therapist with a disability is that I am viewed (by colleagues) as a problem and less able! I would like to see this mindset changed. There needs to be more inclusion in the workplace and increased recognition of both hidden and physical disability challenges; accessibility is not limited to wheelchair access only. It is also deeply important to me that occupational therapists who identify as having a disability are considered equal to all their colleagues, and there is recognition that their lived experiences add to their therapeutic practice and do not detract from it.

Laura Casey, an occupational therapist with cerebral palsy, speaks further about ableism in healthcare:

Being an OT is meaningful for me and an important part of my identity. We are taught as the foundation of our practice to support individuals with meaningful activities. However, it is within occupational therapy, and healthcare more widely, that I have seen a reluctance to include people with lived experience of disability in a sustainable and meaningful way within these professions. For me, this has really opened my eyes to everyday ableism. Our voices are important. Our lived experience is important. We need our voices heard.

Ableism in healthcare, ahh – this is complex, and there are so many questions! Like I said, though, half the battle is realizing that occupational therapists can have disabilities too, and that isn't a problem. We must acknowledge that there are many more professionals out there with lived experience, and this links back to why we need to change the narrative surrounding disability. I'm aware that my cerebral palsy is outwardly noticeable in a conventional, visible way. I am a wheelchair user who has a fairly noticeable lopsided gait and a speech impairment. But I only represent one person with a disability, and the media doesn't often represent the diversity of our community. Disability is diverse, and each individual has their own unique story. We must listen to every word of those unique stories and value every individual's authentic self in order for equity to be achieved.

I will never be able to get rid of the preconceptions that people have. I'm always going to face ableist assumptions and be patronized. It's important that we celebrate winning small battles such as a shop assistant talking to me instead of the person I'm with, as I don't want to become angry at the world. We have to untangle the societal perceptions of those with lived experience of disability and work on this as a collective, no matter what our backgrounds are. Those who work within healthcare need to amplify disabled voices in order to address these issues. Some occupational therapists had never heard of ableism, never mind understanding how to address this. Therefore, the solution is to listen to disabled people.

Writing these final two chapters has been quite hard as I've been trying to think about the bigger picture, forgetting why I'm here in the first place. I'm actually here because I was asked to write a book about my lived experience and authentic stories in order for you to learn and raise questions. Yes, that doesn't dismantle ableism, but it's a start. Disabled occupational therapists are needed and our voices need to be amplified to direct change.

So what's next in my bag of tricks?

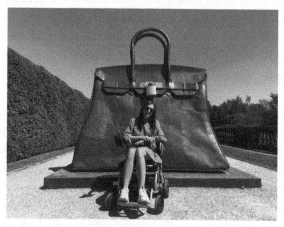

Image 12.1. *Georgia, a white female, sat in her electric wheelchair in a floral dress, outdoors on a sunny day. Behind her is a giant handbag sculpture.*

As much as I love having a goal to work towards to keep me motivated, thinking about my next steps makes me feel overwhelmed. I am so lucky that I get to do what I do. I never thought that four years after starting the blog I began on a whim that I'd be sat here, finalizing my own book. Part of me will never know what the future holds and what my next steps will be, but I certainly want to do more of the work that I am currently doing.

The end goal for me was always to become a paediatric occupational therapist, which is another reason why I enjoy analysing my experiences so much. I mean, I'd love to be a children's occupational therapist one day, but that'll just be the start of another part of my life while I work as a disabled activist and perhaps work towards leadership promotions. I have a lot of career-related goals, and I am looking forward to meeting my current goal of becoming a qualified lecturer in occupational therapy. My work satisfies a lot of my personal qualities and traits, so I love what I do.

My life is not just going to be dedicated to tackling ableism within healthcare or to other research. Yes, I certainly want to work towards my doctorate at some point, which will hopefully be around children, young people and families. I don't know if this will happen any time soon as I also have personal goals to work towards, for example moving out and exploring relationships. I have a lot of internalized ableism around relationships, and recent reflections among friends have made me realize that it's deeper than I thought it was. For example, I want to travel and explore different parts of the world and I'd love to do this with someone. This could be a friend, but it would be nice to think that I could do this with an accepting partner in the future.

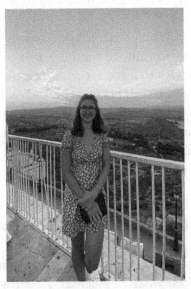

Image 12.2. *Georgia, a white female, stood in a dress with daisies on it and a bag over her shoulder, wearing glasses. She is on holiday abroad, with an epic view and sunset behind her.*

I'm aware that my goals are quite big and won't happen overnight, so I need to start creating and carrying out my action plan. I have avoided working towards these goals in the past, as I know I am going to face many battles and red tape along the way, challenging my mental health. Due to experiencing these problems in the past, being trained in occupational therapy and being heavily involved in disabled activism, I almost know too much. My internalized ableism won't actually stop me achieving these goals. Writing a book and training to become a qualified lecturer are big things that take a lot of energy, but it's now time for me to focus on personal goals. Occupational balance is important after all!

It's important to consider these personal perspectives as we are more than any career we might have. Writing this book has allowed me to focus on how my past affects my future. Even negative experiences or ableism have become pinnacle learning opportunities that I can now utilize in my disabled activism and also feed back to those starting their occupational therapy training. This is why I love guest lecturing – it encompasses every part of me as a disabled person who is also an academic and an activist. Hopefully, this book has also encompassed all aspects of my life. Yes, this narrative stems from my own story, but surely we can use other types of clinical reasoning to generalize and look at this as a macrocosm.

Writing this book has allowed me to identify my own tangible action points as I still have learning to continue. If you have identified any learning that you wish to further, then please do look at the 'Useful Resources' at the end of this book, or expand on your own research. Remember, finishing reading this book is actually the beginning of your own journey towards becoming an anti-ableist ally.

I look forward to seeing how much our collective activism can achieve!

NOT SO TERRIBLE...P.A.L.S.Y. REFLECTIVE LOG
Pausing
Stop and think about what you have read in this chapter. What are your main takeaway points? What are your main questions?

. . . .

. . . .

. . . .

Analysing
Why did this resonate with you?

. . . .

. . . .

. . . .

Learning
What did you learn from this?

. . . .

. . . .

. . . .

Solving
What actions need to be put into place?

. . . .

. . . .

. . . .

Your plan
How will you achieve these actions? What are your goals?

. . . .

. . . .

. . . .

References

Griffiths, S. (2020) 'Ableist attitudes.' *The OT Magazine 37*, Nov/Dec, 22–23.

Griffiths, S. (2020a) 'Occupational therapy and ableism.' *#OTalk*, 18 August. Accessed on 7 April 2023 at https://otalk.co.uk/2020/08/11/otalk-18th-august-2020-occupational-therapy-and-ableism]

Newton, F.M. (2023) *Inclusive PE for SEND Children: A Practical Guide for Teachers.* FB3 Publishing.

Yao, D.P.G., Sy, M.P., Martinez, P.G.V. and Laboy, E.C. (2022) 'Is occupational therapy an ableist health profession? A critical reflection on ableism and occupational therapy.' *SciELO 30*, 1–18. Accessed on 21 September 2022 at https://doi.org/10.1590/2526-8910.ctoRE252733032

Appendix: Reflexivity in Practice Worksheet

Millie Pollitt & Georgia Vine

*Empowered Practice Educator
Conversations chapter author*

Questions to journal/discuss

With the quotes in mind below, consider the enablers and barriers to engagement in occupations (such as the work placement).

Health inequalities research explains that over the last ten years there has been no significant improvement in health outcomes across health inequalities and we are failing those in our community who are most marginalised (Marmot, 2020). The people who are the most marginalised in society exist amongst socio-economic fault lines of gender, race, class, and geographies (Ahmed, Gore, & Langford, 2020). The COVID pandemic has amplified the divide in society causing economic and social ramifications that are far reaching. The impact of inequality is causing unnecessary additional years spent with disability and untimely death (Marmot, Allen, Goldblatt, Herd, & Morrison, 2020). Deaths and disability are avoidable and people working in health and social care have a duty to challenge this (ICF, 2014; RCOT, 2015; WFOT, 2019; HCPC, 2016).

Reflexivity requires the practitioner to "Think about and analyse how their own identity, race, class, sexual orientation, religion, gender and personal circumstance impact on their work and approach" Okitikpi & Aymer (2009)

Disability, according to the 'social model' recognises that the environment can be disabling. "There are many people who don't have a diagnosis or impairment but still face barriers and marginalisation in their access to meaningful occupation, thus, with this lens, also become disabled people." Pollard, Sakellariou and Kroeneburg (2009)

(Hammel, et al., 2015) identified six domains in which a person may experience disabling barriers to participation. These are: Social supports and societal attitudes; Built and natural environment; Assistive technology; Information and technology access; Economic factors; systems, services, & policies & transportation, services, and access.

Reflexive Questions

Can you identify any areas in which your identities intersect to enable or disable your participation?

Which identities provide you with power/privilege? How do you benefit from this?

In which areas do you lack power/are disempowered? Which domains does this show up in?

Do you want support to challenge this?

Thinking about your service user group, can you map their enablers and barriers in access to meaningful occupation?

How will you use your social superpower (post-secondary formal education in largely middle-class institutions of health and social care) to challenge health injustices that service users face?

Food for thought

For example, we know that most occupational therapists are women, about 97% and further it's a largely middle class and white dominated profession. Began (2006) discusses the chasm between the assumed cultural knowledges, values, and practices of those working in largely middle-class institutions of education and healthcare and the experience of the 'other', in this instance she was referring to class but this could be highlighted as any of the other marginalised identities. The experience of trying to fit in, as is explored in the work, is value laden and can be accompanied by shame and stigma. Choosing to self-silence because the individual perceives the listener 'won't get it' is called 'Testimonial Smothering' (Dotson, 2011).

Testimonial smothering is a form of 'epistemic injustice' (Fricker, 2007) or epistemic violence, in this instance referring to the 'choice' to self-silence because it is deemed unsafe for the person to speak up because the listener lacks the capacity to hear a testimony, due to 'pernicious' ignorance.

In other words, it's difficult to begin a conversation about access, rights, the disabling conditions or environment, micro-aggressions, isms in the workplace – if the person, usually in a more powerful position, has the privilege of not having to have had these conversations themselves, especially if the individuals' concerns are prone to being dismissed as unimportant and not part of 'the work'.

Furthermore, this can add on to the experience of burden: epistemic exploitation (Berenstain, 2016). This can be described as: being in a position where you're having to educate people (usually in positions of power who have the capacity to gatekeep) about the experience of marginalisation to negotiate for access to enable your effective participation for which it is a given right to others without the experience of marginalisation. This is also sometimes called referred to as emotional labour. Sometimes people will have legitimate access needs, but wouldn't speak up, because of the additional emotional and physical cost do to so, especially if it is deemed unsafe.

Don't forget

Providing individuals with the space to be heard and seen is a valid and valuable contribution toward practice placement education. The experience of validation (of the barriers or enablers as legitimate access issues) from people in positions of power can be galvanising and can inspire the individual to continue this valuable piece of transformational change work. We know this first-hand as both students and as service users.

Thank you for supporting the future leaders of the profession!

References

Ahmed, N., Gore, E., & Langford, N. (2020, April 30). --Pandemic and Precarity: rethinking what it means to be precarious under covid 19. Retrieved from SPERI Sheffield Political Economy Research Institute: http://speri.dept.shef.ac.uk/2020/04/30/pandemic-and-precarity-rethinking-what-it-means-to-be-precariousunder-covid-19/

Began, B. (2006). Experiences of Social Class: Learning From Occupational Therapy Students. Canadian Journal Of Occupational Therapists, 125

Berenstain, N. (2016). Epistemic Exploitation. An Open Access Journal of Philosophy.

COVID Trauma Response Group. (2020). Supporting Hospital Staff During Covid 19: Early Interventions. Occupational Medicine, 327-329.

Dotson, K. (2011). Tracking Epistemic Violence, Tracking Practices of Silencing. Hypatia, 236-257.

Fricker, M. (2007). Epistemic Injustice: power and the ethics of knowing. Oxford: University Press.

Hammel, J., Magasi, S., Heinemann, A., Gray, D. B., Stark, S., Kisala, P., . . . Hahn, E. A. (2015). Environmental Barriers and Supports to Everyday Participation: A Qualitative Insider Perspective From People With Disabilities. Archives of Physical Medicine and Rehabilitation, 578-588.

HCPC. (2016). Guidance on Conduct and Ethics For Students. London: Health and Care Professions Council.

ICF. (2014). Interprofessional Capability Framework. Sheffield: The Combined Universities Interprofessional Unit.

Marmot. (2020). The Marmot Review Ten Years On. London.

Marmot, M., Allen, J., Goldblatt, P., Herd, E., & Morrison, J. (2020). Build Back Fairer: The COVID-19 Marmot Review. The Pandemic, Socioeconomic and Health Inequalities in England. London: Institute of Health Equity.

Oliver, M. (1990). The Individual and Social Models Of Disability.

RCOT. (2015). Code of Ethics and Professional Conduct. London: College of Occupational Therapists Ltd.

WFOT. (2019). WFOT Position Statement On Human Rights. WFOT.

Acknowledgements

To my parents Glenda and Darron Vine, who certainly faced the most emotional trauma when I was interviewing them. It was hard at times and very emotional, but thank you for being vulnerable with me and for allowing me to add your own authenticity. Another big thanks goes to my sister Matilda, who also allowed me to add and signpost to her raw reflections in the book. It was so important that I encompass my family's views and, to me, it has made the book that more real – thank you!

Margaret Spencer, what can I say? I wouldn't have been asked to write this book if you'd have not been my link tutor on placement. I owe you so much. Thank you for believing in me and for always being there, even when I email you with an idea at 10 pm! I'd also like to thank my friend Georgina Burton who has been helping me put the book together. Thank you for sticking by me during the editing process, even though at times it's taken days to edit one chapter!

Amanda Gaughan, who was also very vulnerable with me and shared feelings and stories that I didn't know about – thank you so much as this allowed me to keep the book current. Of course a big thanks goes to my cousin Tommy; life is definitely better with you! I remember everyone saying that we'd have a special bond – I didn't want to force it, but we definitely do.

A huge thank you to Dr Benita Powrie for your interview and for being so supportive during this whole process. You saw my ideas and helped me to refine them, and I'm so grateful to have worked with you on this. In our professional sphere you have also been a rock to me.

I would also like to thank Dr Mandy Graham, Sam Pywell, Deborah Bergel, Faith Newton, Lee Ridley, Laura Casey, Natalie Hicks, Jeantique Hommel, Devyn Awalt, Jay Webster, and Robyn for providing your insight and allowing me to add elements to the book that aren't just from solely my perspective.

Millie Pollitt, thank you so much for allowing me to share your incredible work, and I can't wait to see what is next for you.

AbleOTUK – we have quite the job on our hands and at times it's tough, but we make up a powerful network and are stronger together! Thanks to Joanne, Michelle, Colette and Anne for all the work you have done in the background. Thanks to everyone who gave me a snippet of their experiences; it really meant a lot to solidify my research and own lived experience.

Thank you to my friends Sophie, Bethany, Libby, Chloe, Ellie and Fran for your friendship, allowing me to share some of our anecdotes and just generally putting up with my loud self. I appreciate all of my extended family, work colleagues and other friends. Whether I met you initially in person or online, you have all allowed me to become more confident as a disabled young woman, and to become the person I am today.

I appreciate everyone who has interacted with my content on social media and my blog. I certainly wouldn't be here if *Not So Terrible Palsy* hadn't taken off! Who would have thought it? Certainly not me!

Last, but by no means least, a big thank you goes to Jessica Kingsley Publishers for believing in me. Writing a book was never something I imagined I could do. Your belief and support has meant so much; I have thoroughly enjoyed this process, and will continue to enjoy working with you in the future.

Useful Resources

Communities

AbleOTUK
Twitter: @AbleOTUK
Instagram: @ableots
Website: https://affinot.co.uk/ableotuk

BAMEOTUK
Twitter: @BAMEOTUK
Instagram: @BAMEOTUK
Website: www.bameot.uk

Chartered Society of Physiotherapy, Diversity networks
Website: www.csp.org.uk/networks/diversity-networks

DisruptOT
Website: www.disruptot.org

LGBTQIA+OTUK
Twitter: @LGBTQIAOTUK
Instagram: @lgbtquiaplusotuk
Website: https://affinot.co.uk/lgbtqiaotuk

Articles

Griffiths, S. (2020) 'Ableist attitudes.' *The OT Magazine 37*, Nov/Dec, 22–23: https://issuu.com/2apublishing/docs/ot_magazine_issue_50_digital_edition

Vine, G. (2020) 'Benefits of online healthcare if one has a disability.' *BMJ Paediatrics Open, Young Voices 4*, 1, 1–2: https://bmjpaedsopen.bmj.com/content/4/1/e000851

Whalley Hammell, K. (2022) 'Editorial: Occupational therapy and the right to occupational participation,' *Irish Journal of Occupational Therapy 50*, 1, 1–2: https://doi.org/10.1108/IJOT-05-2022-031

Yao, D.P.G., Sy, M.P., Martinez, P.G.V. and Laboy, E.C. (2022) 'Is occupational therapy an ableist health profession? A critical reflection on ableism and occupational therapy.' *SciELO 30*, 1–18: https://doi.org/10.1590/2526-8910.ctoRE252733032

Assessments

Autism Queensland, The Family Goal Setting Tool (FGST): https://autismqld.com.au/resources/the-family-goal-setting-tool-fgst

Cerebral Palsy Alliance, What is the General Movements Assessment?: https://cerebralpalsy.org.au/our-research/about-cerebral-palsy/what-is-cerebral-palsy/signs-and-symptoms-of-cp/general-movements-assessment/#:~:text=The%20General%20Movements%20Assessment%20is,age%20(corrected%20for%20prematurity)

Blogs

Chloe Tear: https://chloetear.co.uk
Disabled Travel with Georgina: www.disabledtravelwithgeorgina.com
Life of Pippa: www.lifeofpippa.co.uk
#OTalk: https://otalk.co.uk

Specific blogs

Dickenson, S.-R. (2021) 'What is allyship?' *Communities*, 28 January: www.edi.nih.gov/blog/communities/what-allyship

Inclusive Employers (no date) 'What is allyship? A quick guide.' *Inclusion Allies*: www.inclusiveemployers.co.uk/blog/quick-guide-to-allyship

Pywell, S. (2021) 'The reasonable adjustment/request of dealing in to education: Being an anti-ableist educator in face-to-face classrooms.' *Centre for Collaborative Learning*, 21 October, University of Central Lancashire (UCLan): https://ccl.uclan.ac.uk/2021/10/21/the-reasonable-adjustment-request-of-dialing-in-to-education-being-an-anti-ableist-educator-in-face-to-face-classrooms

Spencer, M. and Vine, G. (2020) 'Experiences of the journey from service user to a professional.' *#OTalk*: https://otalk.co.uk/2020/03/17/otalk-april-21st-april-experiences-of-the-journey-from-a-service-user-to-a-professional

Thomas, D.S.P. (2022) 'Belonging matters.' *AdvanceHE*, 11 October: www.advance-he.ac.uk/news-and-views/belonging-matters

Vine, G. (2021) 'An insight into being the non-disabled sibling: An interview with my sister.' *Not So Terrible Palsy*, 24 September: https://notsoterriblepalsy.com/2021/09/24/an-insight-into-being-the-non-disabled-sibling-an-interview-with-my-sister

Books

Renke, S. (2022) *You Are the Best Thing Since Sliced Bread.* London: Penguin Books: www.penguin.co.uk/books/447975/you-are-the-best-thing-since-sliced-bread-by-renke-samantha/9781529149289

Stacey, P. (2022) *University and Chronic Illness: A Survival Guide.* Barton-upon-Humber: Daisa & Co: www.lifeofpippa.co.uk/product/university-and-chronic-illness-a-survival-guide-by-pippa-stacey

Charities
CP Teens UK: www.cpteensuk.org
Down's Syndrome Association: www.downs-syndrome.org.uk
Positive about Down syndrome: https://positiveaboutdownsyndrome.co.uk
Scope: www.scope.org.uk

Information resources
HCPC (Health and Care Professions Council) (2015) 'Health, disability and becoming a health and care professional' [Booklet]: www.hcpc-uk.org/students/health-disability-and-becoming-a-health-and-care-professional
Health Education England (2022) *Guide to Practice-Base Learning (PBL) for Neurodivergent Students*: www.hee.nhs.uk/sites/default/files/documents/Guide%20to%20Practice-Based%20Learning%20%28PBL%29%20for%20Neurodivergent%20Students.pdfPywell, S., Hicks, N., Vine, G. and Booth-Gardiner, R. (2022) 'Allyship – It's Time to Make It a Meaningful Occupation!' Occupational Therapy Show, 24 November, Birmingham. https://affinot.co.uk/ableotuk/ableotuk-events
Scope (2023) 'Access to Work grant scheme': www.scope.org.uk/advice-and-support/access-to-work-grant-scheme
Werdelin Education (2019) 'Cooperative learning defined: Easy. Efficient. Inexpensive': https://werdelin.co.uk/triple-welcome/cldefined

Reports and government links
DWP (Department for Work and Pensions) (2021) *Disability Confident Employer Scheme.* Collection. London: DWP: www.gov.uk/government/collections/disability-confident-campaign
Equality Act 2010: www.legislation.gov.uk/ukpga/2010/15/contents
GOV.UK (no date) *Access to Work: Get Support If You Have a Disability or Health Condition*: www.gov.uk/access-to-work
GOV.UK (no date) 'Help if you're a student with a learning difficulty, health problem or disability': www.gov.uk/disabled-students-allowance-dsa
Hastings, R. (2014) 'Children and adolescents who are the siblings of children with intellectual disability or autism: Research evidence.' Sibs, University of Warwick: www.sibs.org.uk/supporting-young-siblings/professionals/needs-of-young-siblings/children-and-adolescents-who-are-the-siblings-of-children-with-intellectual-disabilities-or-autism-research-evidence-professor-richard-hasting-2013
HM Government (no date) 'Everything you need to know about student finance!': https://studentfinance.campaign.gov.uk
NHS (National Health Service) (2019) 'Chapter 2: More NHS action on prevention and health inequalities.' In *Online Version of the NHS Long Term Plan*: www.longtermplan.nhs.uk/online-version/chapter-2-more-nhs-action-on-prevention-and-health-inequalities

Videos

BBC News (2019) 'Social media is changing the view of my disability.' 6 March: www.bbc.co.uk/news/41366824

DisruptOT (2022) 'DisruptOT: How it started and how it's going!' May: www.youtube.com/watch?v=AWcwF4FfbOl

Purple Ella (2021) 'Strength Based Support Plans – Disability.' 14 May: www.youtube.com/watch?v=ctJ6KDVy4P8

Young, S. (2014) 'I'm not your inspiration, thank you very much.' TEDx Talk, June: www.ted.com/talks/stella_young_i_m_not_your_inspiration_thank_you_very_much/transcript?language=en

Websites

ARC (Antenatal Results and Choices): www.arc-uk.org

HCPC (Health & Care Professions Council), 'Our commitment to equality, diversity and inclusion': www.hcpc-uk.org/about-us/work-for-us/become-a-partner/our-commitment-to-equality-diversity-and-inclusion

RCOT (Royal College of Occupational Therapists), EDB Insights sessions: www.rcot.co.uk/edb-insights-sessions

Scope, 'Cerebral palsy (CP)': www.scope.org.uk/advice-and-support/cerebral-palsy-introduction

Scope, 'Coming to terms with your child's diagnosis': www.scope.org.uk/advice-and-support/come-to-terms-with-child-diagnosis

Scope, 'Disability Price Tag': www.scope.org.uk/campaigns/extra-costs/disability-price-tag

Scope, 'Disablism and ableism': www.scope.org.uk/about-us/disablism

Sibs: www.sibs.org.uk/about-sibs

UCAS (Universities and Colleges Admissions Service): www.ucas.com